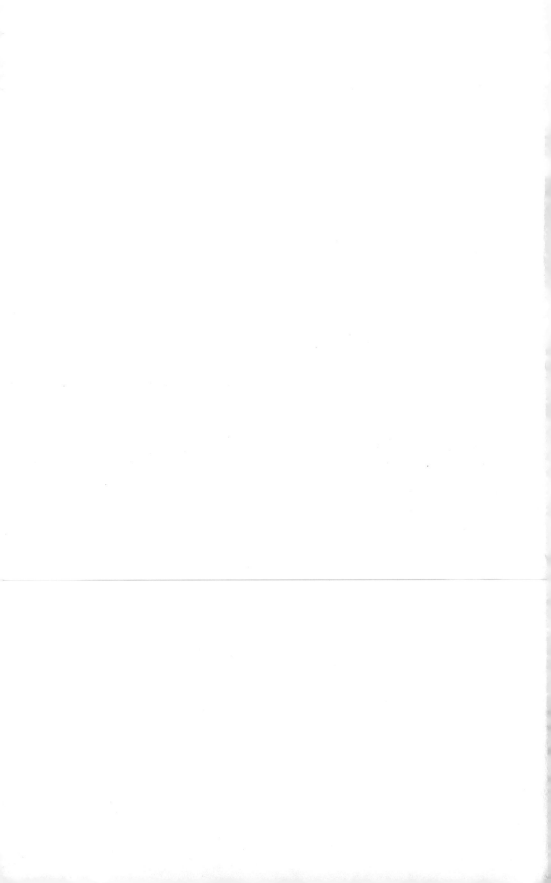

A Field Guide for the Sight-Impaired Reader

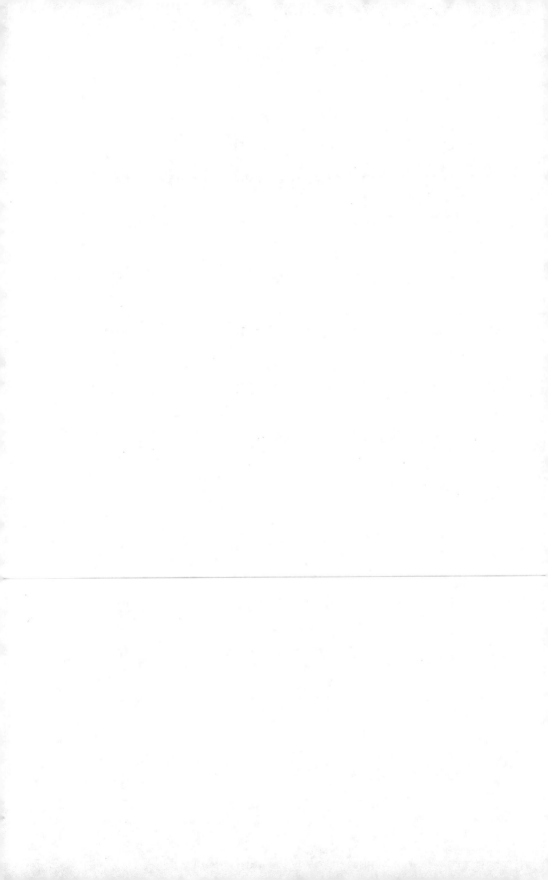

A Field Guide for the Sight-Impaired Reader

A Comprehensive Resource
for Students, Teachers,
and Librarians

Andrew Leibs

Foreword by Richard Scribner

Greenwood Press
Westport, Connecticut • London

Library of Congress Cataloging-in-Publication Data

Leibs, Andrew.
    A field guide for the sight-impaired reader : a comprehensive resource for students,
teachers, and librarians / Andrew Leibs ; foreword by Richard Scribner.
        p.   cm.
    Includes bibliographical references.
    ISBN 0–313–30969–8 (alk. paper)
    1. Blind—United States—Books and reading.   2. Visually
handicapped—United States—Books and reading.   I. Title.
HV1731.L45   1999
011.63—dc21   99–21788

British Library Cataloguing in Publication Data is available.

Library of Congress Catalog Card Number: 99–21788
ISBN: 0–313–30969–8

First published in 1999

Greenwood Press, 88 Post Road West, Westport, CT 06881
An imprint of Greenwood Publishing Group, Inc.
www.greenwood.com

Printed in the United States of America

The paper used in this book complies with the
Permanent Paper Standard issued by the National
Information Standards Organization (Z39.48–1984).

10 9 8 7 6 5 4 3 2 1

For Carolyn Marvin,
who, for hundreds of children,
made the library what it should be:
a place to listen, learn, and laugh

Contents

Foreword

Gaining an education is challenging enough, whether or not an accommodation is required. The more tools you have at your disposal, the better the chances for opening the door to educational and professional success. This book can be a key to opening that door. Within these pages, Andrew Leibs describes a great variety of tools and resources that exist especially for the sight impaired. You will learn about organizations that produce assistive technology for your home, school and office; recorded materials for education or leisure; large print or Braille books; and so on. Throughout the book, you are encouraged to establish your own relationships with vital organizations such as Recording for the Blind & Dyslexic (RFB&D).

When RFB&D was created fifty years ago to help blind World War II veterans take advantage of the GI Bill to earn a college education, books were recorded on vinyl disks that held 12 minutes of material. Imagine how many disks were required to record the complete works of Sigmund Freud! There were not many other options—with a limited number of available Braille books and hired readers—to help a person with a visual impairment gain access to printed materials. Today, the resources available and technologies being developed to assist blind and visually-impaired people are far-reaching and enable you, the student or professional, to achieve every academic goal in preparation for a future full of confident knowledge and unprecedented career potential.

By making a few phone calls, completing the requisite applications and arming yourself with some of the information provided in this book, you can have access to almost any printed materials that you will need or want. Such access will give you the power to handle reading tasks for school or work and will generate possibilities for learning and accomplishments, you may never have had.

The only way to make sure you enjoy all the benefits, of each technological breakthrough and specialized reading service, is to take the responsibility for learning about each one, and then take the steps to bring them into your life. A world of accessible knowledge is out there for you if you know where to find it, and there are many of us along the way to help guide you.

Richard Scribner
President and CEO, Recording for the Blind & Dyslexic

Acknowledgments

I wish to thank several persons for their contributions to this book. In addition to Carolyn Marvin, to whom this book is dedicated, people who read all or part of the manuscript and provided crucial commentary include Alan Ammann, Curtis Chong, Ken Hodkinson, Tom Johnson, Eileen Keim, Gary Mudd, Catherine O'Connor, Heather Hughes, and Dina Rosenberg. In addition, Paula Whitcomb of Recording for the Blind & Dyslexic was an ongoing source of enthusiasm and insight. I also wish to thank Barbara Rader and Debby Adams of Greenwood Publishing Group for their support, candor, and prudent shaping of what is for me a work as personal as it is social.

To the Student

The technology developed to assist the blind can make you the best-read person in your school, and allow you to develop systems for surpassing every academic goal while you use reading to explore your interests and the world in preparation for a future full of confidence and knowledge.

Usually, teachers and administrators talk of special needs, rather than special gifts or advantages, when dealing with sight-impaired students. So early on, you are assigned special teachers who keep you on the compliant path toward graduation, but might not teach you the most precious skill education can foster—the ability to build your own roads—through an introduction to the proper technology and institutions.

This book serves as that introduction. It describes the various tools and resources that exist specially for you, shows the benefits each has to offer, and encourages you to establish your own relationships with vital institutions such as Recording for the Blind & Dyslexic (RFB&D).

With a few phone calls, completed applications, and a little knowledge, you can have access to any book or other written material that you will ever need or want. Such knowledge will give you the power to handle any reading task in school, and will open possibilities for learning and accomplishment you may never have had.

Everything is out there for you: institutions with libraries that are eager to sit you atop the giant earth-moving machines that books become when you use reading to open new roads. The only way to make sure you enjoy all the benefits of each technological breakthrough and specialized reading service is to take the responsibility for learning about each one, and then to take the steps to bring them into your life.

Such steps are little, but the strides they will allow you to make are great. Good luck.

To the Librarian

This book is designed to help sight-impaired students connect with resources that will make them better readers. It carries a simple message: there is a multitude of specialized libraries, services, programs, and organizations that can immediately foster independence and open up a world of reading.

Such a message is easy to post but hard to deliver. That is why this volume is structured to assist you, the librarian. You can be the sea captain of knowledge for students who are often mired in a muddy delta of limited expectations, who may have no one else to help them realize the glorious passages that await.

I hope you will take time to go over this book with any sight-impaired students or patrons you serve, and encourage them to cultivate the many resources that exist specially for them. This book will make you an expert on how to consult with sight-impaired students, their parents, and their teachers on how to find, obtain, and use the various forms of reading aids, such as specially formatted books and adaptive technology that can turn a computer into a multifaceted reading machine.

The book will give you a quick grasp of the workings of the major government and nonprofit organizations, such as Recording for the Blind & Dyslexic and the National Library Service for the Blind & Physically Handicapped. It will help you help students differentiate the many services in order to maximize the immediate benefits each has to offer. The same goes for the State-by-State Resource Guide and the annotated listing of major audio publishers.

Also included are a sample curriculum in specialized format and a Great Books list designed to dramatize the availability in Braille, large print, or cassette of almost any book a student will ever need or want.

What the book ultimately offers is a picture of the true media center for the blind, which is comprised of many libraries, institutions, associated services, and systemized responses. Its front desk is the telephone; its return bin, the nearest mailbox; its shelves, a collection of print and online catalogs reflecting each provider's holdings and focus.

You can help sight-impaired readers by serving as a catalyst for immediate action. Let them make calls to join vital organizations from your phone. Contact some of the Internet sites that contain audio files they can play or download. Help them find readers among your parent volunteers, and make one-time educational use recordings from records in your collection. Any such step can enhance their reading life, and serve as a fitting conclusion to this book.

Last, it should be noted that you can help not only sight-impaired students but also those with learning disabilities: you can remove the stigma associated with auditory reading, and legitimize for students and parents the various reading methods that may be foreign to a student's peers and teachers, but are essential for his or her reading.

Introduction

> When the ear receives subtly; it turns into an eye. But if words do not reach the ear in the chest, nothing happens.
>
> —Rumi

I want to recount some of my experiences as a sight-impaired reader to dramatize this book's singular message: those with visual impairments can create a world of reading equal to that of the fully sighted, provided they learn how to locate, obtain, and use resources and technologies that exist specially for them.

That world of reading is built out of hardware such as tape recorders and computers, and a fluid use of specially prepared resources including recorded books and electronic texts. Sight-impaired students need to learn where these resources come from and how to get them, and to be encouraged to develop their own relationships with institutions to ensure they reap all the academic and personal benefits each has to offer.

Usually, this takes no more than a single phone call to a provider such as Recording for the Blind & Dyslexic or a regional branch of the National Library Service. But too often, such calls are made on behalf of students instead of by them, and so vital connections are never made.

As I look back at the years that took me from junior high

school, when I was pulled under the umbrella of special education, through graduate school and into a career in writing, I am amazed at how the fruits of my reading experience, gathered in 20 years of windfalls, can, with the right mix of information and encouragement, be acquired by a student in an hour or two.

Special technology for reading came to me giftlike, in the same mythic way (or so it felt) that fire was given to ancient man. In third grade, a talking book machine arrived at my house with an assortment of recorded books heavily strapped in black boxes. While I listened to and enjoyed them, there was no spark to light that fire. And no need for it yet, since school reading was more a matter of recognizing and remembering words in class than of using reading to learn.

In sixth grade, two things happened that left a deep imprint on my education, both in terms of how I might succeed and in terms of what others expected of me. In those days, the school had a Huxleyan practice of placing students in groups numbered from 1 to 4, based on intelligence and ability. Based solely on my visual impairment, I was dumped into Group 4. I got the crushing news on the first day of school and imploded with inexpressible shame.

The social studies teacher had done a marvelous thing, however: she had spent an entire summer recording the 900-page Western civilization textbook onto reel-to-reel cassettes. I immediately sensed that I had a leg up on my classmates to compensate for the kneecapping of lowered expectations. I plowed ahead, finishing the book nearly four months early.

THE SPECIAL EDUCATION YEARS

In seventh grade, the guidance office created for me an entire program with special teachers, special courses, and special materials that included books on tape. The guidance counselors placed me in the hands of two special education teachers from the local extension board. Their attack was three-pronged: teach me Braille as a method for reading, teach me typing to transcribe classroom notes on a large-print typewriter, and get me books on tape. Everything looked promising, and I beamed with covetous wonder at the Perkins Brailler, typewriter, and tape recorders that were now mine.

In the fall of eighth grade, after finally getting my first book on tape, and having taken Braille and typing lessons, it was abundantly clear to me what tool was going to drive my education: only tapes would play a significant role. I did not know where they came from, and assumed only teachers could get them. I asked a blunt question at my midyear Individual Educational Plan (IEP) meeting: If I choose to quit the special education classes, can I still get tapes?

At first my teachers said no, because if they were not teaching me, they would have no reason to bring them out. After recognizing my insatiable desire to read, they acquiesced and agreed to provide extracurricular tapes. They said if there was a book I wanted, they would try and get it for me.

I wish I had received more help—for example, that I had been taught the workings of a four-track cassette recorder as a means of note taking, which would have been more useful than typing. Instead, I became engrossed in several novels, but could not understand what happened to half of the book that disappeared between side 2 of tape 1 and side 1 of tape 2 until I accidentally flipped the side selector switch and discovered sides 3 and 4, and the little miracle of each tape being able to house four separate tracks. After that, delight at the freedom and the means to read drove me to devour all the young adult novels long before our English class got to them.

One accomplishment indicative of the precariousness of my reading state came when I read the Richard Adams novel *Watership Down*. When our teacher flagged it as a challenging bit of extracurricular reading, I went to the library to check it out, but my ballooning ambition was burst as the 429-page hardbound book thudded on the counter. I wanted to read the book with my own eyes, but one long afternoon at a pace of five pages an hour told me it wouldn't work. I asked for the tapes, and as soon as they arrived, I plunged in, retracing the 30 pages I'd read, marching into the full sweep of the narrative: through the action, under epigraphs, past stories within stories. But when I'd finished, and was swimming in pride at my accomplishment, one of my relatives was livid. "You didn't *read* it," he sneered, "you *listened* to it."

Was what I had done more like watching a movie? Was it my reading, or someone else's? I knew the story, could answer any question on it, and suspected I would remember details long after fully sighted students whose eyes had scanned every line.

Books are recent inventions compared with the oral tradition that a sight-impaired reader taps into every time the tape or record is playing. Few people finish a book and turn back to page 1 to start again, but technology for the blind makes repeated readings an inevitable pleasure. The eye ushers words into the brain, while the ear is the pathway to the heart, where the best of what we read can live forever. Proper enunciation of phrases and lines that recordings present often impart greater comprehension than the brain can see. In addition, tapes give the confidence to take on what would otherwise be daunting tasks, such as reading *War and Peace*, or going to law school.

INTO POWER

In my senior year, we read some of Shakespeare's sonnets in English class. They were short enough for me to read with my own eyes, but it wasn't until we listened to a recording by John Gielgud that the works came alive, as the proper stresses and enunciation created instant understanding. It was my most powerful experience of the sudden joy and increased comprehension listening can ignite.

When we listened to Paul Scofield as Hamlet rail against Ophelia, a deeper knowledge erupted in me, even if I couldn't decipher meaning in all the phrases. We used recordings to accompany our reading of three Shakespeare plays, and for those few weeks, when auditory reading took center stage, I felt more connected to and enthusiastic about my education than at any other time.

I left high school with no more knowledge of how to get recorded books than when I began, and might never have learned but for a college orientation program for the blind I began a week after graduation. And even there, it was pure chance. That program, in which participants took one college course and received training in study skills, brought me to the Rubicon of my expanding literary goals, and shoved me in. The only course that interested me was American literature, and I set out to read each day's work with my own eyes. Three days in, the tidal bore of dense, difficult, and closely printed pages hit me, and only a desperate use of readers in the following weeks and some marathon sessions with reading lamp and hand magnifier kept me afloat.

TOTAL ACCESS

Late in the summer, I saw another student in the program with RFB (now RFB&D) tapes and, assuming they had been brought by someone else, asked how he got them. He explained how to contact the agency, apply for membership, and use the assigned borrower identification number to order any book, at any time, by myself.

In September, as I began my freshman year at St. John's University, my RFB&D catalog arrived, and instantly became one of the cornerstones of my life. I stress the importance of connecting with Recording for the Blind & Dyslexic because they ask for only your name and proof of disability, and have resources that quickly let you build a reading foundation. RFB&D offers most of the books needed at all education levels, and an efficient use of its full range of services not only increases confidence but also creates a sort of mental triage system for accomplishing all reading tasks.

I could separate reading tasks and assign a solution to each, whether that was a recorded book, a live reader that I paid with reader's aid money from the state department of education, or my own eyes. In my first semester, I read 10 pages a day from the biology text and thus finished the 900-page text in time for finals. Reader's aid paid one roommate to proof my English essays, and another to retype them, and still others, in the large house where I lived for two years, to read chapters in my sociology and history books as I sat contented. My grade point average rose from 2.7 in high school to as high as 3.8 in college, ending with a 3.5.

A deft management of school tasks allowed me to explore other avenues of interest. My mecca of those early college days was the listening room atop the library, where a feast of great works, including every Shakespeare play, and the voices of the world's great authors reading their works awaited me each afternoon. The first day I grabbed *Hamlet* and listened to act III again and again. While biking one October day, I began reciting the scene to myself, and was amazed at the long sections that came out whole through the sheer joy of repeated listenings.

My adult reading life began at the end of my sophomore year in college. It was then that the tools I had begun to use, and a growing list of books I wanted to read, converged into a steady river of reading. That spring, I began stockpiling tapes and books on my kitchen table; there were eight in the first batch, including *The Portable D.H. Lawrence, Candide*, and *The Flowers of Evil*. One by one, I read them, listening long into the night, interrupted only by the tinny rumble of the saucepan boiling water for tea on the gas stove.

I finished college a semester early and devoted much of the nine months before graduate school to expanding my reading in as many ways as I could. I went to my public library to investigate the logistics of talking books, which I had yet to distinguish from RFB&D tapes. I got a new machine, and a smattering of books like the batch that arrived when I was in third grade. This time, however, I learned all the intricacies of the National Library Service system, from where to get my next books (the regional library) to what types of books and materials the system offered.

The selections of best-sellers and classics, all read by professional narrators, enabled me to include contemporary works in my reading, and I enjoyed being able to read popular books that those around me recommended. Avenues of reading for pleasure opened up, and for a time, I reveled in mysteries, rock star biographies, and even romance novels.

Through the National Library Service, I began to receive magazines on flexible disks and noted how cover-to-cover readings became satisfying and easy—another advantage of auditory reading. I also received, through a vocational rehabilitation counselor, a closed-circuit TV that enlarged and clarified print with the twist of a knob. That machine became indispensable for viewing everything from the agate print on sports pages to details in photographs.

Nine years had elapsed since eighth grade when I realized the crucial role recorded books would play in my life at graduate school, where I at last had a solid grasp and supple use of each reading technology, and could create my own independent study projects.

Once you learn how to find and use all resources and technologies, a great thing happens: reading becomes as much a part of you as it is for any fully sighted reader. I know this, and have experienced it through endless satisfying encounters with the written word, whether it was on a languid fall afternoon listening to Agatha Christie stories, the seven months I spent reading the King James Bible, or the week I had to pull together tapes, records, and live readers to finish five novels to write my first book review. If there were boundaries on the extent to which reading could enter my life, I never saw them: not on literary monoliths like *Moby Dick*; on the job, where bibliographic searches turned up many career-building books on writing; or even the whale watch during which I clenched a rail, ignored all jabbering, and, to myself, recited all the songs from Shakespeare's plays.

With this book, you can do in a day what took me 20 years. As Ernest Holmes once said, "A moment's insight is sometimes worth a lifetime of experience." I have had the experience, and I hope this book sparks in you the insight.

A Field Guide for the Sight-Impaired Reader

Chapter 1: The Foundation Resources

This chapter profiles the major resources with which a sight-impaired person builds a world of reading. Though you may already use materials from such institutions as Recording for the Blind & Dyslexic or the National Library Service, establishing your own personal relationship is the surest way to derive the maximum benefits each has to offer.

These resources are the eternal library cards, the life changers, the points of departure on the road of reading. Or, in the case of advocacy-focused organizations such as the National Federation of the Blind, they provide the road maps to other vital institutions and opportunities. As you join these and other organizations (a simple process you can initiate today), and make contact with the professionals there, you will discover resources that exist just for you, and people who are eager to help you see the world through reading.

All cassette books produced by these agencies contain four tracks (sides) that play at a reduced speed and require a Library of Congress or compatible tape player that you can obtain from your state's National Library Service affiliate or from a variety of vendors and institutions.

So make the calls, request the applications, provide answers and documentation, and get connected now. If your school already secures materials for you, that's fine. But those are few books, compared with the whole libraries that belong to you.

RECORDING FOR THE BLIND & DYSLEXIC

Your house of knowledge has no pillar more secure than Recording for the Blind & Dyslexic (RFB&D), which puts a library of over 80,000 recorded books for every phase of education, and an array of recording and research services, a computer or phone line away.

RFB&D developed in the late 1940s as a hub of volunteer initiatives to record textbooks for blind and disabled veterans attending college after World War II. Education is still its main focus, though its services have become more diverse and far-reaching.

At the heart of RFB&D is the C. V. Starr Master Tape Library, which adds about 4,000 new titles each year. RFB&D's national network of volunteers assiduously combs educational publishing at all levels to produce crucial texts as soon as possible, and will usually readily record any book you request for free, provided the book falls within the educational scope of the library and you mail them two print copies.

These two services alone can take all reading-related stress out of high school or college and level the playing field with the fully sighted. With your membership, you can order all necessary books for an upcoming class or school year in minutes, a process that will allow you to see what books might need to be recorded or obtained in other formats. You will be able to read books one or more times over the summer prior to classes, and reread them with ease.

RFB&D's reference staff will also do bibliographical searches that can provide you with computer or mail-delivered printouts or direct mailings of books in subject areas of special interest to you, whether for a research paper, on-the-job training, or pleasure reading.

Such services make setting and achieving goals instantly possible, and give you a higher gear of enthusiasm, born of access, that will allow you to maneuver easily and comfortably through each phase of your education.

Other services include a growing library of electronic texts or E-texts, which are books stored on computer disks that can be read with either a word processor or a speech synthesizer. This format is ideal for reference books. Imagine using the fast-forward button on a tape recorder to look up a word in a 50-cassette dictionary. A computer query retrieves it instantly.

Membership requires only the completion of an application, documentation of disability (such as a signed note from a low vision specialist), and payment of a registration fee, after which you will receive a borrower identification number that speeds the ordering process. RFB&D also charges an annual user fee. Both fees should be paid by your school, which purchases and provides textbooks for all sighted students without charge.

The fastest way to get a book is to call RFB&D Customer Service with the title and author. Books are copied from master tapes and shipped within two weeks either in blue plastic boxes (for books with six cassettes or fewer) or in corrugated boxes. You can keep books up to a year. To return them, flip the address card underneath the plastic box, or tear off your half of the address label on the corrugated box, then drop the container into a mailbox. There is never any postage charge to receive or return books; both are covered by the Free Matter for the Blind provision of the Postal Service.

You can purchase RFB&D's two-volume catalog or use the electronic version on its website. Both are powerful tools: the catalogs instantly show the preponderance of materials, and can lead you to new areas of interest; the on-line database returns instant answers.

Recording for the Blind & Dyslexic

Headquarters	20 Roszel Road Princeton, NJ 08540
Phone	609–452–0606
Toll free	800–221–4972
Reference librarian	609–520–8031
Internet	www.rfbd.org
Audio library	80,000 titles with educational focus
Other formats	Electronic text (E-text) reference books
Fees	$25 per year plus a one time $50 registration fee
Services	Recording service, bibliographic searches, scholarships, sells selection of portable and desktop four-track tape players
Eligibility	Anyone unable to read standard print due to a visual impairment, learning disability, or other physical disability
Application process	Return completed application with disability documentation for immediate membership
Established	1948, in New York City

THE NATIONAL LIBRARY SERVICE FOR THE
BLIND & PHYSICALLY HANDICAPPED

While RFB&D is your one-stop shop for educational texts and references, the National Library Service for the Blind & Physically Handicapped (NLS) helps readers build on that crucial base by providing a steady stream of popular literature (best-sellers as well as classics), recorded periodicals, braille books, as well as permanent loans of all necessary equipment.

NLS is where you go for the books you want to have read, such as *Middlemarch* or *Ulysses*, and for those you want to read, like Anthony Robbins seminar retreads, diet books, and Star Trek novels. It's all here, from the *Meditations* of Marcus Aurelius to John Lennon's interview in *Playboy*. In July 1998, the NLS recorded talking books numbered 46,000.

While RFB&D monitors educational trends, NLS watches the *New York Times Book Review* and the *Washington Post Book World*, so if a book is in the news, you will likely find it in *Talking Book Topics*—a bimonthly publication highlighting the latest NLS books—soon thereafter.

NLS uses professional narrators, so its recordings are of a very high quality, which can augment one's reading pleasure and comprehension. The late Alexander Scourby, longtime voice of the National Geographic specials on PBS, read nearly 500 books, including the entire King James Bible.

The other major NLS holding is its collection of roughly 10,000 braille books, which, like cassettes, can be borrowed for a year. Since state libraries within the NLS system share resources, and copies of individual braille titles tend to be scarcer than tapes, obtaining a book might take a few weeks.

The NLS membership process begins like that of RFB&D, only this time you call the network library for your state (see listing in Appendix A) to request an application. After submitting the completed form with documentation of disability, you will receive a phone call or letter, at which time you can verify information and select playback equipment (talking book record and cassette players, headphones, etc.). Your library will usually send a selection of books and catalogs along with the machines to get you started.

Catalog themes range from all talking books produced in the past year to more specific collections, such as mysteries, romances, and books for young adults.

At that point, you are free to read. However, you should know about two policy quirks.

First, you might want to pass on the option to have the library select books for you and send them automatically. When someone other than you selects the books, you don't always receive books on subjects you enjoy.

Second, let your librarian know that you wish "on demand" rather than "turnaround" service. "On demand" means your order is filled immediately. On "turnaround" (the default policy), you ask for eight books, they send you whichever titles are available, then more titles as you make returns. This can be confusing and frustrating, especially if you want to keep books for additional readings. And if you read *Cassette Books—1997* and mailed in the form to order 20 books, there's no telling which ones will come first. You may go bookless for two months, then find 12 on your doorstep. All obstacles between wanting a book and having the tapes can be erased by calling in your order and requesting immediate action.

NLS books are copied from master recordings and sent to each regional library, where your order is filled. Unlike RFB&D, which fills all orders from master recordings, NLS books are finite in number. If a book is not on the shelf of your regional library, you may have to wait. If it is an important book for school, you should tell your librarian, who can usually secure a copy through interlibrary loan.

National Library Service for the Blind & Physically Handicapped

Headquarters	1291 Taylor Street, NW Washington, DC 20542
Phone	202–707–5100
Toll free	800–424–8567
Internet	lcweb.loc.gov/nls
Audio library	60,000 books with focus on popular fiction, nonfiction, and classics
Other formats	Large selection of braille books; over 70 popular magazines; vast music materials collection
Services	Free permanent loans of playback equipment
Eligibility	Anyone unable to read print due to a physical or learning disability
Application process	Return completed application with disability documentation to your regional library (see Appendix A)
Established	1931, by act of Congress

To return a book, flip the address card and drop the book in a mailbox.

The NLS also offers a wealth of popular and professional magazines on cassette and record, as well as in braille, large print, and computer diskette. Magazines are a powerful and often underused resource that can sharpen reading habits, boost overall knowledge, and fill in another corner of your reading tapestry. Cover-to-cover reading of a publication, something rare among fully sighted readers, often occurs easily and automatically for readers listening to tapes. Magazines available include *Analog Science Fiction/Science Fact, Backpacker, Sports Illustrated* (including *SI for Kids*), *Smithsonian*, and *Playboy* (braille only).

For the musically inclined, a collection of over 30,000 items, including braille and large-print scores and instructional recordings, awaits you.

THE AMERICAN PRINTING HOUSE FOR THE BLIND

Since 1858, the American Printing House for the Blind (APH) has produced special materials for blind readers. Since the 1879 passage of the Act to Promote the Education of the Blind, it has received federal funding to keep up the good work.

APH offers approximately 1,500 books in braille (in addition to those it produces for the National Library Service) and 5,200 in large print. These are vital resources, especially in areas such as mathematics and foreign languages, which demand a more immediate sense of what's on the page.

You don't join APH; you buy its resources. The easiest way to do that is to call or write to request copies of its two main catalogs, one featuring books, the other, products. With the 396-page *APH Catalog of Accessible Books for People Who Are Visually Impaired* on your shelf, and an eye on upcoming reading requirements, planning requests that you can submit to your school or vocational rehabilitation department will be easy.

In addition, APH offers a wealth of products related to the education of the blind, including every type of reading machine and text enlarger, braillewriters and all associated supplies, tactile maps and globes, and items for daily use such as clocks, watches, and key chains. Such an emphasis on day-to-day needs is pushing APH away from its pure educational focus. The goal is to make every written thing (company memos, romance novels, utility bills) accessible to the blind, whether through braille or other technologies.

One of APH's greatest assets is a cutting-edge piece of technology called Louis, a massive on-line database that lets you search the holdings of over 200 organizations that provide materials for blind readers, including RFB&D and the NLS. Named for Louis Braille, Louis should be your first stop in the material-gathering phase of each school year. The database can be accessed free of charge through the APH website.

Another service APH offers is the on-demand production of large-print books. Just as RFB&D will record any book, APH can create a customized large-print copy. Two clean copies of the book are required. Copyright permission is handled for you, and the book is completed and mailed in one to two months. Currently there is a charge of 25 cents per page.

The American Printing House for the Blind

Headquarters	1839 Frankfort Avenue Louisville, KY 40206
Phone	502–895–2405
Toll free	800–223–1839
Fax	502–899–2274
Internet	www.aph.org
Audio library	Records books for the National Library Service
Other formats	Sells wide selection of braille and large-print books
Services	On-demand creation of large-print books; maintains Louis, an on-line database of alternative format books; provides *Newsweek* and *Reader's Digest* on cassette; sells complete line of adaptive products
Eligibility	Materials may be purchased by anyone
Established	1858

NATIONAL ASSOCIATION FOR VISUALLY HANDICAPPED

Another major source of large-print books is the 7,000-volume collection at the Robert L. Fastie Memorial Library, maintained by the National Association for Visually Handicapped (NAVH). The collection has an NLS feel to it, giving the sight-impaired a wealth of pleasure reading, including popular novels, celebrity biographies, and memoirs. It also contains every blindness-related book the NAVH publishes.

Though this library might only serve as the airport newsstand in your world of reading, joining NAVH can, through its newsletters, website, and phone consultations, keep you abreast of important developments, including companies offering new programs and services, the latest medical news related to blindness, and free referrals to low vision centers and other resources.

NAVH has a long commitment in working with manufacturers to develop and test products to aid the partially sighted, including a large button adapter for a TV remote control. It also publishes a catalog that features over 200 items, from magnification and illumination devices to large-print playing cards.

NAVH holds seminars at its New York headquarters and

National Association for Visually Handicapped

Headquarters	22 West 21st Street
	New York, NY 10010
Phone	212–889–3141
Fax	212–727–2931
Internet	www.navh.org
Audio library	2,000 recorded books
Other formats	8,000 large-print books
Services	Field tester and developer (with manufacturers) of visual aids; comprehensive source on latest sight-related medical research
Membership	Annual fee of $40 includes mailing of all library materials
Established	1954

---

its San Francisco office. The organization also runs a "fun room" in New York where patrons can test and be trained on every conceivable piece of low vision equipment, as well as receive counseling and support.

NATIONAL FEDERATION OF THE BLIND

Through its Materials Center, the National Federation of the Blind (NFB) offers over 1,200 pieces of literature—pamphlets, banquet speeches, books, and reports—that focus on every legal and social aspect of blindness. As with NAVH, it also sells products used by the blind in education and daily life.

If you ever feel isolated as a blind person, sense you are not being treated fairly, are concerned about an issue related to blindness (such as travel or accommodations), need copies of federal laws and regulations in all formats, or want to network with blind students or professionals in various fields, the NFB, with chapters in every state, can provide confidence-building, action-taking information. The NFB keeps an eye on everything.

"What Should a Library for the Blind Be?," "Rehabilitation Act Reauthorized—Victory for the Blind," and "On Becoming a Wise Consumer of Low Vision Services" are among the 600 pieces of free literature available. An area of particular strength is braille education and advocacy, which the NFB promotes through books (e.g., *The Bridge to Braille Reading* and *School Success for the Young Blind Child*), and through initiatives such as the Braille Mentoring Project and maintenance of resources like the Braille Transcription Resource List, which profiles all distributors, publishers, and on-demand transcribers of braille.

Another vital reading service developed by the NFB is

the Newsline for the Blind Network™, comprised of recordings of local and national newspapers that blind persons access over the telephone. The service electronically synthesizes the complete text of the *New York Times*, the *Chicago Tribune, USA Today*, and many local newspapers, which can all be searched and read from a touch-tone phone, anywhere, at any time—another example of reading technology that begins with facilitation and ends with extension.

NFB also runs the International Braille and Technology Center for the Blind (IBTC), which houses the world's most comprehensive collection of adaptive technology for the sight impaired, including braille embossers, translators, refreshable displays, printers, and speech synthesizers. IBTC also publishes reviews of new devices. Anyone can visit the center (located at its national headquarters in Baltimore) by appointment. The IBTC also manages NFB NET, an Internet bulletin board for networking, downloading issues of *The Braille Monitor* and other NFB publications, and testing new computer technology.

Three more programs should be noted. The NFB, in conjunction with the U.S. Department of Labor, runs Job Opportunities for the Blind, a national office that publishes a cassette job-hunting bulletin eight times per year and maintains a reference and referral program. The NFB also awards annual scholarships totaling $88,000 to top students enrolled in postsecondary education programs. Lastly, NFB has divisions devoted to endeavors, professions, or academic pursuits ranging from industrial work to music to teaching.

National Federation of the Blind

Headquarters	1800 Johnson Street Baltimore, MD 21230
Phone	410–659–9314
Fax	410–685–5653
Internet	www.nfb.org
Library	Publishes, resells, and distributes special format books and literature on the social aspects of blindness though its Materials Division
Services	International Braille and Technology Center for the Blind, Newsline talking newspaper, Job Opportunities for the Blind, special interest division, unparalleled braille advocacy
Eligibility	Blind or visually impaired
Established	1940

AMERICAN FOUNDATION FOR THE BLIND

Established in 1921, the American Foundation for the Blind (AFB) is a leading resource and advocacy force for blind persons in the United States. This is the organization that Helen Keller—the most influential blind crusader in history—helped build up through over 40 years of work in government relations and international diplomacy.

For the sight-impaired reader, the AFB's most direct benefit is the recording it produces for the National Library Service in its state-of-the-art studios. In 1986, in an effort to recognize and perpetuate the high quality of NLS recordings, the AFB instituted the Alexander Scourby Narrator of the Year Awards, named for the most popular talking book narrator of all time.

On the AFB website, readers can listen to the most recent award ceremony in its entirety, as well as search through the organization's offerings of free literature on virtually all aspects of blindness, read through back issues of its newsletter and press releases, and order materials from the AFB Press.

The AFB Press is a leader in the areas of blind education, mobility, and access. It publishes the *Journal of Visual Impairment & Blindness*, the field's most influential publication, as well as reference books, especially the comprehensive *Directory of Services for Blind and Visually Impaired Persons in the United States and Canada*, which features many resources, including all low vision centers and guide dog schools in each state, that are beyond the scope of this book.

Another solution-oriented service AFB provides is the Careers & Technology Information Bank (CTIB), a national network of blind and sight-impaired individuals throughout the United States who use assistive technology and are willing to share their experiences with others. Finding such a person in your state and spending 20 minutes on the phone might be the fastest way to connect with crucial services in your area.

AFB maintains a toll free information line anyone can use to receive counseling or referrals on any aspect of blindness.

Like the NFB, the AFB is a storehouse of information that includes the M. C. Migel Library, the world's largest collection of materials related to blindness, and the massive Helen Keller Archive, in which you can retrace the steps of her long and extraordinary journey, from being received by Queen Victoria to corresponding with Albert Einstein and Franklin D. Roosevelt, and being awarded the Presidential Medal of Freedom by Lyndon Johnson. Anyone can view the archive by appointment, and much can be viewed or read on AFB's website.

Keller traveled the world, corresponded with the greatest men and women of her age, and was a powerful advocate for the blind, whether she was addressing Congress in support of legislation or elevating, with the weight of her personality and tireless effort, the federation that became her lifelong cause. AFB is still widening the roads of acceptance and opportunity her life's journey so steadfastly constructed. One way it accomplishes this is by presenting annual awards, named for Keller, to those whose achieve-

---

American Foundation for the Blind

Headquarters	11 Penn Plaza Suite 300
	New York, NY 10001
Phone	212–502–7600
Toll free	800–232–5463
Fax	212–502–7777
Internet	www.afb.org
Library	Produces talking books for NLS; the AFB Press publishes wide range of books on blindness, as well as the *Journal of Visual Impairment & Blindness* and other periodicals, pamphlets, and videos
Services	Runs the Careers & Technology Information Bank (CTIB), a mentoring network; maintains the Helen Keller Archives and the M. C. Migel Memorial Library, the world's largest print collection of blindness materials
Established	1921

---

ments have improved the lives of the blind. Recent winners include such luminaries as Ted Turner, for advancing descriptive audio in films, and 3M chairman Livio D. De-Simone, for an ongoing program to hire and train blind workers.

The resources profiled above should provide you with most of the reading material you will need as a student. While they might lack the time and marketing resources to find you, the contact you initiate will put you on their mailing lists and in their databases. Through their newsletters, brochures, and websites, you will be kept informed about new technology, services, scholarships, and books as they become available.

A good first step for obtaining a desired book is to consult the Louis database on the American Printing House for the Blind website. If you do not have Internet access, call their toll free number and ask them to run a search for you. Since Louis contains all titles available though Recording for the Blind & Dyslexic and the National Library Service, chances are your search will end with immediate success. Then you can simply call the right institution to order the book, using its shelf or cassette number.

If a title is not available, take immediate action to have it produced for you in the format you desire. Recording for the Blind & Dyslexic will record most books (two clean copies required), and the American Printing House for the Blind will enlarge any book for a quarter a page. A listing of braille transcribing services appears in the next chapter, in which we will start to build on this foundation by discussing additional resources available in each of the specific formats, including braille and large print, and where to obtain all the tools with which to use them.

Chapter 2: Technology Resources

This chapter describes the technological aids specifically designed to increase the sight-impaired student's ability to read. Such tools, from small hand-held magnifiers to closed-circuit televisions and computers that can be turned into personal reading systems, are what truly level the metaphoric playing field of literacy on which the blind and fully sighted strive. These tools are indispensable, and the sight-impaired reader must become aware of and have access to all devices that can make reading more efficient.

Along with descriptions of the most popular types of reading aids, this chapter provides manufacturer contact information. Visit their websites; order and read their catalogs; get on their mailing lists; make them aware of you. If you do not know what tools are available, you will be unable to specify to special education teachers or vocational rehabilitation counselors (who will do most of the buying for you) the exact items that can most positively impact your life through reading.

School librarians, who deal with hardware and software vendors more regularly than students or parents, can be especially helpful in specifying the most appropriate and cost-effective equipment. They also may allocate part of their annual audiovisual hardware and software budget for equipment that benefits the disabled. Since schools retain and later recycle (often through the library) items purchased on behalf of special needs students, the librarian should be consulted on all purchases.

FOUR-TRACK TAPE PLAYERS AND RECORDERS

Cassette books produced by the National Library Service and Recording for the Blind & Dyslexic cannot be played on standard tape players. To maintain their special copyright agreements with publishers, books are recorded and circulated only to individuals who possess the necessary playback equipment. The tapes play at the slower speed of 15/16 inch per second (ips) instead of the standard 1 7/8 ips, and are recorded onto four tracks (sides) rather than two.

The National Library Service makes four-track cassette players and talking book machines (which play flexible disk recordings of magazines) available to all eligible readers through each state's network library (see Appendix A). In addition, recorders manufactured by commercial companies are often purchased for students as part of a special education plan or by a vocational rehabilitation department.

Sight-impaired readers should maintain at least three cassette players. Though the NLS will send out a new machine if one breaks or is damaged (you must pack and return the original), going even a day without access to books can ruin midterm exam preparation or disrupt a good read. Also, just as the fully sighted can read in any room of the house, on the bus, or in the park, you should enjoy the same opportunities by having players in your room, at school, and in your backpack at all times.

Cassette player-recorders come in many shapes and sizes, from library models that accommodate six pairs of headphones to mini boom boxes and units indistinguishable from a Sony Walkman. All such devices will play standard cassettes in addition to NLS recordings. Prices vary from about $70 to $300, depending on features. A free NLS pamphlet profiles the leading manufacturers, of which three popular ones are mentioned below. In addition, Recording for the Blind & Dyslexic, the American Printing House for the Blind, and the American Foundation for the Blind resell four-track machines.

Innovative Rehabilitation Technology, Inc.
1411 West El Camino Real
Mountain View, CA 94040
Phone: 415–961–3161
Toll free: 800–322–4784

Possibilities: *TTRS-145*, modified Sony that plays on four tracks, records on two, and has AM/FM radio, est. $149.95; *TTP-112*, modified Aiwa player, est. $79; *TTR-165*, a mini boom box featuring AM/FM radio and weather band, est. $154.

LS&S Group
PO Box 673
Northbrook, IL 60065
Phone: 800–468–4789
Internet: www.lssgroup.com

Possibilities: *Tape Talker*, a Walkman-like unit that, at est. $59.95, is the least expensive four-track player available; *Ultimate*, a mini boom box with AM/FM stereo sound, est. $169.95; *Educorder*, a library unit with six headphone jacks, est. $239.95.

Maxiaids
PO Box 3209
Farmingdale, NY 11735
Phone: 516–752–0521
Toll free: 800–522–6294
Internet: www.maxiaids.com

Possibilities: *Sony Dream Machine*, a clock radio with AM/FM stereo featuring power backup, est. $139.95; *modified Aiwa Superbass* stereo with four-track play, two-track record, est. $129.95; *Panasonic Hands Free Library of Congress tape transcriber*, est. $369.95.

CLOSED-CIRCUIT TELEVISIONS

Closed-circuit televisions (CCTVs) are magnification devices that consist of a sliding tray, camera, and monitor. Reading material is placed on the tray under the camera, and the images, which can be enlarged up to 100 times, depending on the system, and which the reader can manipulate in a variety of ways, are cast onto the monitor mounted above. CCTVs can also be used as computer monitors, often giving readers a larger screen and greater visual flexibility over screen enlargement software programs.

CCTV controls are easy to use: a flip of a switch turns black words on a white background into high-contrast white on black, which some readers find more visually appealing. Color monitors may cast yellow letters on a blue screen. Magnification, focus, and contrast are set and changed with the turn of a knob.

With a CCTV, a sight-impaired reader has access to all the small but vital objects in literacy's junk drawer, such as bus and railway timetables, classified ads, appliance instructions, loan applications, insurance policies, and prescriptions. CCTVs also enhance the viewing of postcards, photographs, and maps.

Some students live on their CCTV, while others complain of stiff necks and vertigo from watching the words of their book atop the gliding tray sway and swirl on the screen as they maneuver up and down the pages. Readers need to run their own tests to make up their minds. A good way to do this is to call local libraries, many of which now have CCTVs, and once one is located, go there with various types of reading materials. One might also call the manufacturers to set up a meeting and demonstration with the salesperson covering your region.

CCTVs are expensive: a black-and-white unit with a 14" monitor costs about $1,800. Color units start at around $3,000. Vocational rehabilitation will often include a CCTV as part of the computer package it normally purchases for college-bound students. The two foremost companies making CCTVs are Optelec and Telesensory Corporation. Their units are largely similar in terms of features and functionality. Most CCTVs are stationary, weighing approximately 40 pounds. A portable option, popular among librarians, is manufactured by Innoventions, Inc. The Magni-Cam is a lightweight camera and magnifier system that can turn any TV into a CCTV. It can also be used with a head-mounted display (resembling a large pair of sunglasses) or a portable, 25-ounce, flat-screen monitor.

Optelec US, Inc.
6 Lyberty Way
Westford, MA 01886
Phone: 978–392–0707
Toll free: 800–828–1056
Internet: www.optelec.com

Possibilities: *2000 monochrome magnifier* with 17" monitor, est. $1,795; *Clearview color video magnifier* with 17" monitor, est. $3,545; *Spectrum Super VGA computer-compatible camera* (no monitor), est. $3,095.

Telesensory Corporation
520 Almanor Avenue

Sunnyvale, CA 94086
Phone: 408–616–8700
Toll free: 800–227–8418
Internet: www.telesensory.com

Possibilities: *Aladdin Reader*, 14" monochrome monitor, est. $1,749; *Aladdin Rainbow*, 14" color monitor, est. $2,995; *Aladdin Genie*, with color selection and computer compatibility, est. $2,995.

Innoventions, Inc.
5921 S. Middlefield Road, Suite 102
Littleton, CO 80123
Phone: 303–797–6554
Toll free: 800–854–6554
Internet: http://www.magnicam.com/magnicam/index.htm

Possibilities: *Magni-Cam electronic magnifier*, est. $695; head-mounted display system, est. $1,200; flat-screen display system, est. $1,200.

PERSONAL COMPUTERS

The personal computer (PC), whether it's an IBM-compatible or Macintosh system, is becoming the technological hub of the sight-impaired reader's life, affording the ability to create, manipulate, store, and retrieve texts that can then be translated into a reader's preferred format. A computer will read a book to you; enlarge any document, application, or web page; and make braille reading more flexible by allowing you to quickly print documents or load them into a portable note-taking device.

The increasing power and integration capabilities of the computer continue to transform reading technology. For example, reading machines used to be stand-alone devices that converted scanned text into simulated human speech, such as the Kurzweil Reader, introduced in 1977. Since the technologies that machine deployed (scanning, character recognition, and speech synthesis) can be performed on a PC using a scanner, speech synthesizer, and specialized software, most development trends in reading technology are aimed at the computer. As RFB&D and the NLS begin to digitize their tape libraries for access over the Internet, the computer will become even more central to the sight-impaired reader's life.

Computers change so drastically in price and power from month to month that a discussion of specific systems and models one should purchase is impractical here. If you are sight-impaired, and plan to attend college or take professional training, a computer will usually be purchased for you by the state department of vocational rehabilitation (see Appendix A). This will often be an IBM-compatible computer, which tends to be more useful to the sight-impaired than the more visually oriented Apple Macintosh family.

Any system purchased for you by a school or vocational rehabilitation counselor will usually come with the appropriate adaptive programs and accessories, including a speech synthesizer, screen reader, scanner, large monitor or CCTV, and various braille devices (described in greater detail in Chapter 4).

SPEECH SYNTHESIZERS

Speech synthesizers began as physical devices that were attached to a computer and worked in conjunction with software to allow users to hear keyed-in letters and commands identified audibly. Today, many synthesizers are software programs that utilize a system's embedded sound cards and external speakers, though external models still

exist. One of the most popular models is DECtalk, produced by Digital Equipment Corporation, which comes in
several versions, including PC-based software and a portable unit that attaches via a serial port to any computer.
DECtalk is also embedded in many software reading programs.

Most synthesizers contain a variety of voice personali-
ties, both male and female, so users can select a style and
tone that appeal to them. Each voice's pitch can be ad-
justed.

Once this virtual voice box is installed, the linear eyes
of screen-reading software can bring words to life on any
given screen. This is protean technology indeed: some operating systems, screen readers, and peripherals include
speech synthesizers (a growing trend), and some do not. If
you desire to read using a computer, be sure the proper
software and the means to listen (sound card, speakers)
come with your system.

Digital Equipment Corporation
VMS Group
153 Taylor Street
Littleton, MA 01460
Phone: 800–344–4825
DECtalk PC. System requirements: CPU, 286 or higher;
RAM, 20 KB, hard drive space: 1 MB. Price: est. $1,195.

Humanware, Inc.
6245 King Road
Loomis, CA 95650
Phone: 800–722–3393
Internet: www.humanware.com
Keynote GOLD speech synthesizers. Models include the
Stand-alone, est. $995, *PC-card*, est. $795, *PCMCIA type II*

card for notebook computers, est. $1,150, and the *Keynote Companion* est. $1,995, a personal organizer that also functions as an external synthesizer.

SCREEN READERS

Screen readers do what their name suggests: they read aloud all decipherable words on any given screen, whether in a word-processing document, spreadsheet, database, or Internet site. Screen readers automatically read all information under the mouse as it moves, as well as the selections in menus and each option in a dialogue box. Most have user-definable cursor tracking keys and "hyperactive" windows that let users monitor the screen for specific occurrences, such as text matches.

Screen readers work with all operating systems, and are especially useful in web browsing. Most support all the major speech synthesizers, but do not contain them. If you have separate reading software such as Kurzweil 1000 or Open Book (see below) that reads scanned text or imported files, you will still need a screen reader for text in all other types of files.

Henter-Joyce
11800 1st Court North
St. Petersburg, FL 33716
Phone: 800–336–5658
Internet: www.hj.com

JAWS 3.2 for Windows. System requirements: CPU, 386 or higher; RAM, 4 MB; hard drive space, 20 MB. Operating system: Windows 3.1, 95, or 98 and MS-DOS. Price: est. $795. Note: JAWS for DOS 2.31 became freeware on January 1, 1999, and can be downloaded from the company's website.

GW Micro, Inc.
725 Airport North Office Park
Fort Wayne, IN 46825
Phone: 219–489–3671
Internet: www.gwmicro.com

Window-Eyes, Version 2.1. System requirements: CPU, 386 or higher (Pentium recommended); system: Windows 3.1X with 4 MB of RAM, or Windows 95 with 8 MB of RAM (16 recommended). Price: est. $595.

SOFTWARE READING PROGRAMS

Since most PCs now ship with built-in sound cards and external speakers, one can turn a computer into a reading system with a flatbed scanner and a reading software program. Kurzweil once made stand-alone reading machines; now it makes software, as do Arkenstone and Telesensory. Most programs do more or less the same thing—recognize and read aloud text that is scanned into the computer or imported from a word-processing file.

Users control the basic functions—scanning, reading, and stopping—with the keyboard.

Kurzweil 1000 contains a 175,000-word dictionary, has a selection of 14 distinct reading voices, and allows background scanning, on-screen text enhancement for visual reading, and word-processing functions. Telesensory's program Reading AdvantEdge™ has virtually the same features. Open Book from Arkenstone accomplishes many of the same functions for a lower price, but requires that users already have a speech synthesizer, such as DECtalk.

Though the three programs can read any scanned text or imported word-processing document, none replaces the more comprehensive screen-reading programs like JAWS, produced by Henter-Joyce, which can recognize windows, buttons, and menus, and is thus the key tool for web browsing.

Kurzweil Educational Systems, Inc.
411 Waverley Oaks Road
Waltham, MA 02454
Toll free: 800–894–5374
Internet: www.kurzweiledu.com

Kurzweil 1000 Version 3.0. System requirements: CPU, Pentium; system, Windows 95/NT; RAM, 32 MB; CD-ROM drive; sound card and speakers; TWAIN compatible scanner. Price: est. $1,095 with Flextalk speech synthesizer; est. $1,295 with DECtalk speech synthesizer.

Telesensory Corporation
520 Almanor Avenue
Sunnyvale, CA 94086
Phone: 408–616–8700
Toll free: 800–227–8418
Internet: www.telesensory.com

Reading AdvantEdge™. System requirements: CPU, 133 MHz or higher; system: Windows 95; RAM, 16 MB; hard disk space: 50 MB; SoundBlaster 16 card or compatible; speakers; CD-ROM drive; scanner; Adaptec 2910 B SCSI controller card or DMA compatible. Price: est. $995.

Arkenstone
555 Oakmead Parkway
Sunnyvale, CA 94086–4023
Phone: 800–444–4443
Internet: www.arkenstone.org

Open Book, Version Three. System requirements: CPU, 486 or higher, minimum 20 MHz; system: MS-DOS 6X or 5X, Windows 95 or 3.1; RAM: 16 MB recommended; hard disk space:

25 MB; scanner; speech synthesizer (many supported, including DECtalk PC, Accent, and Sounding Board). Price: est. $995.

READING MACHINES

Despite the computer's co-opting of speech-based reading technology, read-only machines such as Telesensory's Expert Reader (what the Kurzweil Reader became after two corporate acquisitions), and the Arkenstone VERA (Very Easy Reading Appliance) still have their uses, especially in libraries and among persons who need reading more than computer access.

These machines, as easy to use as tape players, consist of a processing unit with a scanning surface on which reading material is placed, and a small, attached keypad that allows readers to scan, read, and stop with simple precision. Some units have additional features: the latest VERA offers an optional display screen for large-print viewing of scanned text.

Arkenstone
555 Oakmead Parkway
Sunnyvale, CA 94086–4023
Phone: 800–444–4443
Internet: www.arkenstone.org
   VERA (Very Easy Reading Appliance). Price: est. $2,995.

Telesensory Corporation
520 Almanor Avenue
Sunnyvale, CA 94086
Phone: 408–616–8700
Toll free: 800–227–8418
Internet: www.telesensory.com
   Aladdin Ambassador Pro. Price: est. $3695.

SCREEN MAGNIFICATION SOFTWARE

Screen magnifiers are software programs that allow computer users to magnify text and graphics on a screen exponentially with one keystroke. Most programs can magnify a screen from 2 to 20 times its original size. Two popular magnification programs are listed below. Demo disks can be downloaded from each of their websites, or by calling the company.

Ai Squared
PO Box 669
Manchester Center, VT 05255
Phone: 802–362–3612
Internet: www.aisquared.com
Zoom Text XTRA Level 1. Requirements: Windows 95 or 3.1, 486 processor or higher, and 8 MB of disk space. Price: est. $395. *Zoom Text for DOS*. Requirements: DOS 3.0 or higher, 85K of free memory, and VGA graphics adapter. Price: est. $295. *Zoom Text XTRA Level 2* is an integrated magnifier and screen reader. Price: est. $595. *Zoom Text XTRA Level 3* (under development) will add OCR, scanning, form handling, and printing.

Henter-Joyce
11800 1st Court North
St. Petersburg, FL 33716
Phone: 800–336–5658
Internet: www.hj.com
MAGic 2.0 for Windows. Requirements: CPU, 386 or higher, running Windows 95/98 or 3.1X with 4 MB of RAM, 650K hard disk space, and 256 color display. Price: est. $349. MS/DOS version, est. $349. Windows/NT version, est. $995.

HANDHELD MAGNIFIERS

Some readers with a fair amount of vision can read using just their reading glasses; others, with glasses and the aid of a small magnifying glass. Every company or institution that sells low vision products carries an array of handheld magnifiers in every shape, size, and power; some with lights, some with bifocals (a small, higher-powered lens contained within a larger one), some pocket-sized, and some with stands.

The same goes for reading lamps—another vital tool for sight-impaired readers—as well as talking watches and calculators, canes, plastic signature and check writing guides, and recreational items from braille dominoes to large-print playing cards.

It is hard to know what little item might add a sizable level of convenience or joy to one's life, so take the time to explore, remembering that the companies listed below and others in this chapter will not find you. You have to contact them.

Independent Living Aids, Inc.
27 East Mall
Plainview, NY 11803
Phone: 800–537–2118

The Lighthouse, Inc.
Product Center
36–02 Northern Boulevard
Long Island City, NY 11101
Phone: 800–829–0500

Maxiaids
PO Box 3209
Farmingdale, NY 11735

Phone: 516–752–0521
Toll free: 800–522–6294
Internet: www.maxiaids.com

Science Products for the Blind
PO Box 888
Southeastern, PA 19399
Phone: 800–888–7400

Chapter 3: Braille Resources

The development of braille in the nineteenth century is undoubtedly the most significant event in the history of blind literacy and education. It seems, however, that no sooner had Louis Braille created the language of raised dots—modified from an earlier system called "night writing"—than debate began regarding the language's viability and proper place in the world of blind people. Braille eventually supplanted every other embossed language or lettering system introduced over the past 175 years, but it is still locked in a battle to establish itself as the primary source of learning among blind people.

Today, braille has both ardent champions and a host of blind persons with no interest in learning or using the language. The availability of cassettes or talking books offers what some regard as a more convenient way to read, and many who lose their sight later in life find it difficult to begin learning a new language. Also, an ongoing effort to create a Unified Braille Code has sparked further division among braille readers, whose numbers have shrunk steadily since the 1960s.

That no blind person had any hope of becoming literate and educated before the existence of braille often goes unmentioned.

Braille is the only component in the lives of many blind people that affords genuine literacy—the ability to read words directly on a page, to encounter and grasp the topology of texts, to write and read what you have written, and to have complete communicative freedom—and therefore its availability must be assured and broadened.

Like any language, braille is easiest to learn in childhood, and can be fully mastered only if it is practiced in all phases of life, from class reading and reading for pleasure to letter writing, note taking, and a fluid use of the language as a way of seeing the world. A key question a young student must answer early on, with the help of parents and teachers, is whether braille will be essential for overall literacy and learning.

This is not an easy question to answer; it is deeply personal, and many outside factors must be weighed, including the availability of braille teachers, a supportive atmosphere in school, and the proximity of resources—not just books and educational tools, but also seasoned braille users who might serve as mentors.

According to Curtis Chong, Director of Technology for the National Federation of the Blind, two things are needed to become a competent braille reader: immersion in braille in all phases of education, and complete access to materials in braille. In elementary school, Chong points out, sighted students receive daily reading instruction, and reading skills are fostered in every phase of learning. A blind student learning braille may get only two classes per week.

Getting equal education is your legal right and your responsibility. This chapter lists many of the resources that braille readers need to develop competence in the language.

BRAILLE EQUIPMENT

The essentials for communicating in braille are paper and a means to write in the language, such as a braillewriter or slate and stylus. Such items, as well as various accessories, can be purchased from a sources that include the American Printing House for the Blind and the National Federation of the Blind. Usually these items are initially provided by the special education programs in public schools.

Though braille users do most of their writing on a brailler, advances in computer technology afford greater flexibility in creating, transferring, printing, and storing of documents.

Using a personal computer, a blind student now has the option to create documents with a word processor and speech synthesizer, and convert the text into Braille using translation software such as MegaDots or Duxbury. If a scanner and optical character recognition (OCR) software are integrated into the system, any written document can be loaded into the computer to be read aloud using a screen reader, or converted into braille.

Once in braille, documents can be printed out using a braille embosser, or read using a terminal with a refreshable display, an electronic device connected to the computer that uses small pins to create braille characters along a fixed line of braille cells. One line is displayed at a time, which the reader "refreshes" by using a directional key or cursor routing function. In addition, computer-generated documents or electronic texts can be downloaded into portable note-taking devices such as a Braille Lite, which contains a standard braille keyboard, a speech synthesizer, and a refreshable display. Such technology offers flexibility and enhanced opportunities for bringing braille into all phases of education. It is, however, expensive. In some cases, equipment may be purchased as part of a special education program or later through the vocational rehabilitation department of your state.

Following is an introductory list of braille products and where to obtain them. A more comprehensive listing can be found on the National Federation of the Blind website: www.nfb.org/aas.htm.

Braille Writing Devices

For manual writing of braille onto paper.

The Perkins brailler
Howe Press of Perkins School for the Blind
175 North Beacon Street
Watertown, MA 02172–9982
Phone: 617–924–3490
Internet: http://perkins.pvt.k12.ma.us/index.htm
Perkins manual brailler, est. $640; *electric brailler*, est. $900.

The NFB brailler
Materials Center
National Federation of the Blind
1800 Johnson Street
Baltimore, MD 21230
Phone: 410–659–9314
NFB also sells slates, styluses, and a variety of braille papers. Prices: aluminum pocket slate (4-line, 27-cell), est. $18; plastic pocket slate, est. $3 (a stylus is sent with each new slate); pencil-shaped stylus with pocket clip and braille eraser, est. $7.50; 400 sheets of heavyweight paper, est. $10.

Braille Terminal

Attaches to computer and displays text as braille on re-freshable display.

Alva braille terminal
Humanware, Inc.
6245 King Road
Loomis, CA 95650
Phone: 800–722–3393
Internet: www.humanware.com

Company sells two portable and two desktop versions. The desktop versions offer refreshable lines of 45 or 85 eight-dot cells. Prices range from $3,995 to $11,995.

Translation Software

Converts normal word-processed or scanned English into braille.

Duxbury braille translator (for Windows or MS-DOS)
Duxbury Systems, Inc.
435 King Street
PO Box 1504
Littleton, MA 01460
Phone: 978–486–9766
Internet: world.std.com/~duxbury

System requirements for Windows version: CPU, 386 or higher (486/66 or faster recommended); RAM: 4 MB; hard drive space, 6 MB; Microsoft Windows version 3.1 or 95. Price: est. $595. For MS-DOS version: CPU, 286 or higher; RAM, 2 MB; hard drive space, 4 MB; MS-DOS version 3.3 or higher. Price: est. $550.

MegaDots (version 2.0)
Raised Dot Computing
408 South Baldwin Street
Madison, WI 53703
Phone: 800–347–9594
Internet: www.rdcbraille.com

System requirements: CPU, 386 or higher (486 recommended); RAM, 8 MB; hard drive space, 15 MB; Price: est. $540.

Speech Synthesizer

Converts computer commands and text into speech.

DECtalk PC2 speech synthesizer
Compaq Computer Corporation
Digital Product Sales
153 Taylor Street TAY2–2/G6
Littleton, MA 01460
Phone: 800–344–4825
System requirements: CPU, 286 or higher; RAM, 20 KB; hard drive space, 1 MB. Price: est. $1,195.

Screen Reader

Converts all on-screen words, including websites, into speech.

JAWS for Windows (version 3.2)
Henter-Joyce
11800 1st Court North
St. Petersburg, FL 33716
Phone: 800–336–5658
Internet: www.hj.com
System requirements: CPU, 386 or higher; RAM, 4 MB; hard drive space, 20 MB. Windows 3.1, 95, or 98 and MS-DOS. Price: est. $795. *Note*: JAWS for DOS 2.31 became freeware on January 1, 1999, and can be downloaded from the company's website.

Braille Embosser

Printer.

Romeo classic braille embosser
Enabling Technologies
1601 Northeast Braille Place
Jensen Beach, FL 34957
Phone: 800–777–3687
Internet: www.brailler.com
Prices: Romeo embosser (25 CPS), est. $2,555; same unit with single-sheet option, est. $2,855; basic unit with ET Speaks, which echoes entered commands, est. $2,755; Romeo embosser with ET Speaks and single-sheet option, est. $3,055; Romeo embosser (40 CPS), est. $3,555.

Portable Braille Devices

Stores braille for output through speech or refreshable display.

Braille 'n Speak
Braille Lite
Blazie Engineering
105 E. Jarrettsville Road
Forest Hill, MD 21050
Phone: 410–893–9333
Internet: www.blazie.com
Features: Each Series 2000 model has Perkins-style braille keys for easy note taking; word-processing functions including spell check, a talking clock, calendar, and phone book; and ample storage space for notes or reading on the go. The Braille Lite has an (18-cell display) Prices: Braille 'n Speak 2000, est. $1,299; Braille Lite 2000, est. $3,395.

MAJOR PUBLISHERS OF BRAILLE BOOKS

As discussed in Chapter 2, the National Library Service for the Blind & Physically Handicapped is the largest single source of braille books, with approximately 10,000 titles. The NLS contracts with several organizations, such as the Clovernook Center in Cincinnati and the American Printing House for the Blind, to publish the books it distributes. Other publishers, such as the National Braille Press, seek to fill reading needs not addressed by the NLS, such as best-sellers, cookbooks, and computer titles, more quickly.

American Printing House for the Blind
1839 Frankfort Avenue
PO Box 6085
Louisville, KY 40206
Phone: 502–895–2405
Internet: www.aph.org
    In addition to its work for the NLS, the APH has a catalog featuring approximately 1,500 braille titles that is free upon request.

Braille International
3290 Southeast Slater Street
Stuart, FL 34997
Phone: 407–286–8366
Internet: www.gate.net/~braille/
    The William A. Thomas Braille Bookstore stocks over 1,000 titles. A braille or print catalog is available upon request.

Clovernook Center
Opportunities for the Blind
7000 Hamilton Avenue
Cincinnati, OH 45231

Phone: 513–522–3860
Internet: www.clovernook.org
A name and organization to know, offering many products, programs, and services. Heavily involved with braille magazine production and the sale of customized paper products.

Label Specialties
8014 Vinecrest Avenue
Louisville, KY 40222
Phone: 502–425–3136
Braille and cassette labels.

National Braille Press
88 Saint Stephen Street
Boston, MA 02115
Phone: 617–266–6061
Internet: www.nbp.org
Publishes popular titles on variety of subjects, and also transcribes requested books for a fee. Offers Braille Book of the Month Clubs for children and adults.

Seedlings
PO Box 51924
Livonia, MI 48151–5924
Phone: 800–777–8552
Internet: www.seedlings.org
Nonprofit organization that has a selection of over 300 braille books for preschool and elementary readers.

SELECTED BOOKS ON BRAILLE LITERACY

Beginning Braille for Adults
By Ramona Wahlof
National Federation of the Blind
Includes braille manual with instructional cassette. Price: est. $4
1986. 29 pp.

Braille Literacy: Issues for Blind Persons, Families, Professionals, and Producers of Braille
By Susan J. Spungin
American Foundation for the Blind
Softcover: pack of 25, est. $50; braille: free single copy offered
1990. 12 pp.

The Bridge to Braille: Reading and School Success for the Young Blind Child
By Carol Castellano and Dawn Kosman
National Federation of the Blind
Diskette or large print. Price: est. $12
1997. 191 pp.

Foundations of Braille Literacy
By Evelyn J. Rex, Alan J. Koenig, Diane P. Wormsley, and Robert L. Baker
American Foundation for the Blind
Print or braille: est. $36.95
1995. 153 pp.

Guidelines and Games for Teaching Efficient Braille Reading
By Myrna R. Olson in collaboration with Sally S. Mangold
American Foundation for the Blind
Softcover: est. $23.95
1981. 116 pp.

Handbook for Learning to Read Braille by Sight
By Leland Schubert
American Printing House for Blind
Paperback: est. $25.20
1966. 85 pp.

The McDuffy Reader: Braille Primer for Adults
By Sharon Duffy
National Federation of the Blind

Braille (without print), est. $15; print (dot formations pictured), est. $15; cassette, est. $10
1989. 76 pp.

Reading by Touch
By Susanna Millar
Routledge
Hardcover: est. $85; softcover: est. $24.99
1997. 352 pp.

PERIODICALS

There are many magazines and newsletters available in braille, and many that discuss issues surrounding braille literacy, such as technological developments and recent legislation. Some are available through NLS, and you should request a copy of their publication *Magazines in Special Media*, which also profiles magazines available through other sources.

AFB News. Newsletter chronicling activities of the American Foundation for the Blind, a leading organization in braille advocacy and publishing. Frequency: semiannual; cost: free; available formats: cassette, large print; publisher: American Foundation for the Blind, New York City, 800–232–5463.

BVA Bulletin. Newsletter of the Blinded Veterans Association; includes news on technology, legislation, employment, and association activities. Frequency: bimonthly; cost: free; available formats: cassette, large print; publisher: Blinded Veterans Association, Washington, DC, 800–669–7079.

Braille Book Review. Announces new braille books produced by the National Library Service, and updates additional library services. Includes recorded version of *Talking Book Topics*. Frequency: bimonthly; cost: free; available formats: braille, computer diskette, electronic access, large print; publisher: National Library Service. Request from regional library.

The Braille Forum. Chief publication of the American Council of the Blind, covering organizational activities as well as technology, legislation, and human interest stories. Frequency: monthly; cost: free; available formats: braille, cassette, computer diskette, electronic access, large print; publisher: American Council for the Blind, Washington, DC, 800–424–8666.

Braille Mirror. One of a few magazines offering selected readings from national magazines and newspapers with columns of interest to blind readers. Frequency: 10 issues per year; cost: free; available format: braille; publisher: Braille Institute of America, Los Angeles, 800–272–4553.

Braille Monitor. The voice of the National Federation of the Blind, covering legislation, recent legal cases, and social concerns related to blindness issues. Also features new technology and programs, as well as human interest stories. Frequency: monthly; cost: est. $25 per year, or free upon request; available formats: braille, cassette, electronic access; publisher: National Federation of the Blind, Baltimore, 410–659–9314.

Dialogue. Articles, poems, and stories by and about blind individuals; news; columns on education, employment, sports, and daily living. Frequency: quarterly; cost: est. $28 per year; available formats: braille, cassette, large print; publisher: Blindskills, Inc., Salem, OR, 800–860–1224.

Expectations. Anthology of excerpts and chapters from books recommended for children ages 8–13. Includes embossed pictures and a scratch-and-sniff section. Frequency: annual; cost: free; available format: braille; publisher: Braille Institute of America, Los Angeles, 800–272–4553.

The Matilda Ziegler Magazine for the Blind. General interest articles from national publications, including poems and short stories, sections devoted to readers' letters and special notices, and an editor's column highlighting blindness-related developments. Frequency: monthly; cost: free; available formats: braille, cassette; publisher: The Matilda Ziegler Magazine for the Blind, New York City, 212–242–0263.

NBA Bulletin. Voice of the National Braille Association, discusses topics related to braille and audiocassette transcribing. Frequency: quarterly; cost: est. $30 per year, free to NBA members; available formats: braille, cassette, computer diskette; publisher: National Braille Association, Rochester, NY, 716–427–8260.

Syndicated Columnists Weekly. Collection of columns on a wide range of topics, including economics, politics, social issues, and sports, by America's foremost syndicated columnists. Frequency: weekly; cost: est. $20.80 per year; available format: braille; publisher: National Braille Press, Boston, 617–266–6160.

Tactic. Computer magazine for the sight-impaired, featuring the latest in adaptive technology and a readers' forum. Frequency: quarterly; cost: est. $25 per year; available formats: braille, computer diskette, large print; publisher: Clovernook Center, Cincinnati, OH, 513–522–3860.

Tapping Technology. Comprehensive look at technological devices, services, and products to assist persons with disabilities. Frequency: quarterly; cost: free; available formats: braille: cassette, computer diskette, large print; publisher: Tapping Technology, Baltimore, 800–832–4827.

The World Blind. Multilingual publication (English, French, Spanish) discussing blindness-related topics, such as rehabilitation, in the international community. Frequency: biannual; cost: free; available formats: braille, cassette; publisher: World Blind Union, Avenue Bosquet 58, 75007 Paris, France.

BRAILLE TRANSCRIPTION SERVICES

Many organizations, as well as individuals, will for a fee translate printed matter into Grade II braille, thus answering, however slowly, a reader's need for many types of materials. Forms, shorter documents, and business cards can be embossed in about a week; a full-length book might take a year. Most charge between 15 and 30 cents per Braille page, with additional setup and binding fees. Normally, text is scanned into a computer and converted into braille using a translation program such as MegaDots or Duxbury. Pages are then printed out using a braille embosser, bound, and mailed out. Some translators accept computerized documents only. A more complete list can be found on the National Federation of the Blind website: www.nfb.org.

Associated Services for the Blind
919 Walnut Street
Philadelphia, PA 19107
Phone: 215–627–0600
Will transcribe from print or IBM disk (est. 50 cents per page, est. $2 per page for music, math, and computer-related material). All work is proofread.

Braille Institute
741 North Vermont Avenue
Los Angeles, CA 90029–3594
Phone: 213–663–1111
Will braille anything but music from print or IBM disk. Price and turnaround time varies with job.

Braille Line, Incorporated
3901 North Vincent Avenue
Peoria Heights, IL 61614

Phone: 309–686–0855

   Price quotes free on request.

Dancing Dots
130 Hampden Road Third Floor
Upper Darby, PA 19082–3110
Phone: 610–352–7607
Internet: mccannw@netaccess.com

   Specializes in braille music technology. Lime or MIDI file, est. $3.25 per page, print score, est. $4.75 per page, setup, est. $20 per hour (charged by quarter hour, minimum $5).

Guild for the Blind
180 North Michigan Avenue Suite 1700
Chicago, IL 60601
Phone: 312–236–8569

   Preference is given to work-related transcription (cost: est. 25 cents per braille page). Turnaround time varies. Materials accepted in print or on disk. Additional charge (est. $3) per volume for binding and covers.

Massachusetts Association for the Blind
Attention: Braille Department
200 Ivy Street
Brookline, MA 02146
Phone: 617–732–0249

   Will transcribe at a rate of est. 15 cents per page for individuals.

Naperville Area Transcribing for the Blind (NATB)
670 North Eagle Street
Naperville, IL 60563
Phone: 708–963–0944

   Call for pricing and formating information.

National Braille Association, Incorporated
3 Townline Circle

Rochester, NY 14623–2513

Phone: 716–427–8260

Cost: transcription est. 35 cents per page if ordered from agency; est. $1 per volume for binding.

Sun Sounds

3124 East Roosevelt

Phoenix, AZ 85008

Phone: 602–231–0500

Can produce braille, large-print, computer disk, or audio materials. Documents can be scanned, typed in, or received on disk or via modem. Cost: est. 30 cents per page, less for large orders. Turnaround time: three weeks or less. No music or Nemeth type (used for scientific and mathematical braille).

Volunteers for the Visually Handicapped

8720 Georgia Avenue Suite 210

Silver Spring, MD 20910

Phone: 301–589–0894

Cost: est. $18 per hour and est. 20 cents per braille page; no interpoint, Nemeth, or music. Binding fees included. Accepts material on disk only.

BRAILLE ON THE INTERNET

As with every other subject these days, you can find information about braille on the Internet more quickly than anyplace else. A great jumping-off point is a list of sites on the New York Institute for Special Education History website, which can be found at www.nyise.org/braille.htm. Legislative initiatives, Louis Braille biographies, the history of reading codes for the blind, and a more extensive listing of products, advocacy organizations, and resources can be accessed starting there. Another portal to that ocean of information is on the Enabling Technologies website (www.brailler.com), which has a links page offering information on braille history, translation, products, shareware, and toys.

Chapter 4: Large-Print Resources

There are a growing number of agencies providing materials in large print. In some cases, these constitute an efficient method of bridging learning between the world of unaffected vision and that of the sight-impaired.

While listening to cassettes might be an easy way to read, it does not let the reader directly encounter text and graphics—the act that teaches topography, grammar, and spelling, and also opens up the joy of experiencing words and images on a page. Just as with braille, large print can be the tool that transforms the mechanics of language into literacy.

Large print, however, does some of its best work with graphical elements: the bold labeling of a triangle, the decipherable contours and place-names on an enlarged map, the elongated and legible loops in a diagram of a kidney, the spelling variations in the neat rows of a French verb conjugation. Large print lets sight-impaired readers possess the knowledge locked in these images, which in a normal classroom setting might be lost to them.

Readers can use large print as a means for experiencing written material as completely as possible. This can be done by obtaining books and magazines in large print, having materials enlarged by a specialty publisher, asking a teacher to provide you with an enlarged photocopy of all materials used in a class, and creating your own large-print materials using either a personal computer or the local copy shop. There are also tools that enlarge text, from simple hand held magnifiers, to closed-circuit televions, to software programs that, with a keystroke, let computer users expand or contract the size of images displayed on the screen.

There are many ways to get a closer look at that which creates knowledge, so explore as many as you can.

MAJOR LARGE-PRINT BOOK PUBLISHERS

Large-print book publishing has increased steadily in the past decade, as the baby boomers pass into middle life and are susceptible to a condition called presbyopia, a hardening of the eye lens. A glance at available large-print titles suggests a softening of the desire to learn, as the genres of escapism dominate. The sight-impaired reader, the secondary target audience in large-print publishing, may take pleasure here, but will find little help for high school or college. The American Printing House for the Blind and on-demand large-print publishers are the best source for that. As with any other product that might enhance your education, do not let cost be an obstacle—work the items into your special education or vocational rehabilitation plan.

The American Printing House for the Blind
1839 Frankfort Avenue
Louisville, KY 40206
Phone: 800–223–1839
Internet: www.aph.org
Has a selection of approximately 5,000 large-print titles, including high school and college textbooks, and classic fiction and nonfiction.

Bantam-Doubleday-Dell
Customer Service
2451 South Wolf Road
Des Plains, IL 60018
Phone: 800–223–5780
Internet: www.bdd.com
Publishes large-print editions of mainstream adult novels.

Thomas T. Beeler
PO Box 659
Hampton Falls, NH 03844
Phone: 603–772–1175
Beeler Large Print publishes 24 new titles per year, all hard-cover, in 16-point font. The company also publishes Sagebrush Large Print westerns, and resells many books by other publishers on a variety of topics, including popular fiction and nonfiction, and Cyber Classics, classic paperbacks in large print.

Chivers North America
PO Box 411
5131 Lafayette Road
Hampton, NH 03842–0015
Phone: 800–621–0812
Internet: www.chivers.uk.com
Wide selection of fiction and nonfiction titles in both large print and audio.

Doubleday Large Print Home Library
Membership Service Center
6550 East 30th Street
Indianapolis, IN 46206
Phone: 317–541–8920
A large print book of the month club comprised of an introductory deal (often four books for a dollar) and a commitment to buy four more books in the next two years.

North Books
PO Box 1277
Wickford, RI 02852
Phone: 401–294–3682

Small but strong selection of popular fiction and classics, all hardcover and in 16-point font.

Random House
400 Hahn Road
Westminster, MD 21157
Phone: 800–726–0600
Internet: www.vintagebooks.com

Major publisher offers many popular large-print titles (16-point type), especially best-sellers.

Thorndike/G. K. Hall Press
PO Box 159
Thorndike, ME 04986
Phone: 207–948–2962
Toll free: 800–223–1244

Thorndike and G. K. Hall, both Macmillan imprints, publish mainstream fiction and nonfiction, including westerns, romances, and biographies.

Transaction Large Print
Rutgers—State University of New Jersey
35 Berrue Circle
Piscataway, NJ 08854
Phone: 888–999–6778
Internet: www.transactionpub.com

Transaction's far-reaching backlist contains over 300 titles, including fiction, biography/autobiography, contemporary history, health and self-improvement, and animals and nature. Transaction also resells ISIS Books, which features classic British and American literature.

Ulverscroft Large Print Books
PO Box 1230
West Seneca, NY 14224–1230
Phone: 800–955–9659
Internet: www.ulverscroft.co.uk

Popular fiction and nonfiction: mysteries, romance, westerns—in both hardcover and paperback—with many titles aimed at young adults.

MAJOR RESELLERS OF LARGE-PRINT BOOKS

Amazon.com
1516 Second Avenue, Fourth Floor
Seattle, WA 98101
Phone: 206–622–2335
Internet: www.amazon.com

Resells virtually any available book through its website, usually at reduced prices. The site has a powerful search engine and a secure server with which users can order (with a credit card) any of 2.5 million titles.

The Large Print Bookshop
PO Box 5375
Englewood, CO 80155
Phone: 303–721–7511
Internet: users.aol.com/largeprint

Sells over 1,000 large-print titles new, used, and ex-library editions; has fiction, nonfiction, and classics; sells through its store in the Denver Mall and by mail order. Free catalog available through website.

LARGE-PRINT LIBRARIES

Besides the public library in your town and its growing list of large-print titles, two libraries circulate books nationally to sight-impaired readers.

National Association for Visually Handicapped
22 West 21st Street
New York, NY 10010
Phone: 212–889–3141
Internet: www.navh.org

The Robert L. Fastie Memorial Library, maintained by the National Association for Visually Handicapped in New York, has over 7,000 books, most of which are donated by mainstream publishers, but also include all NAVH books and materials on blindness. Annual membership fee for unlimited library usage is est. $40.

Wisconsin Educational Services Center for the Visually Impaired
1700 West State Street
Janesville, WI 53546
Phone: 608–758–6146

Wisconsin Educational Services Center resells large-print titles published by the American Printing House for the Blind, does on-demand book production, and circulates educational books used in Wisconsin schools to anyone who requests them.

ON-DEMAND LARGE-PRINT BOOK PRODUCERS

The following agencies will produce a large-print copy of any book, charging per-page enlargement and book binding fees—usually in the area of 50 cents per original page. Readers obtain and submit a copy (sometimes two copies are required) of the desired book, and the agency obtains copyright permission from the publisher. Turnaround time is usually from four to eight weeks. Unless otherwise directed, agencies enlarge the entire book, from title page to the last index entry, so you might wish to have them skip certain pages to reduce the overall cost. Enlarging photographs sometimes lessens resolution, but sight-impaired readers will appreciate the increased ease of reading graphics such as maps, charts, and diagrams.

Large Print Books
1951 West 38th Street
Casper, WY 82604
Phone: 307–577–6389
Internet: www.starcomfg.com/books.html

LRS (Library Reproduction Service)
14214 South Figueroa Street
Los Angeles, CA 90061
Phone: 800–255–5002
Internet: www.lrs-largeprint.com/index.htm

Volunteer Transcribing Services
205 East Third Avenue Room 207
San Mateo, CA 94401
Phone: 415–344–8664

DO-IT-YOURSELF ENLARGING

Making print bigger, and thus easier to read, is yet another solution in an ongoing effort to read one's way through the world. A handheld magnifier used in conjunction with reading glasses is a good start. A better one is to acquire a closed-circuit television, which will enlarge anything set under its camera up to 100 times. These items, and the best places to purchase them, are found in Chapter 3. If these items are to be specifically purchased for you (the ideal situation), do not hesitate to research devices on your own so you can recommend the exact equipment you prefer.

The computer, whether IBM or Macintosh, can, if equipped with the right hardware and software, allow you to create your own large-print documents.

Obviously, anything that you write with a word-processing program can be enlarged by selecting the text and changing the point size (a point is 1/72 of an inch high). Standard text (the default on many word processors) is 12 points. Large-print publishers use 14, 16, 18, and, very rarely, 24-point type. You can enlarge letters to as much as an inch in height (72 points), though this would yield fewer than 20 words on each printed page. At that rate, *The Great Gatsby* would take up 3,000 pages.

As well as personal documents written from scratch, you can enlarge books, articles, and other reading material by scanning pages into the computer, running them through an optical character recognition (OCR) program that converts word images into text, importing the file to the word processor for enlargement, and then printing the final document. The process—which requires a flatbed scanner and OCR software—is more practical for shorter documents, such as an essay or article handed out in class.

A faster, though costlier, method for book enlargement is on copiers at the local print shop, where two pages at a time can be enlarged up to four times the original size.

Whether you enlarge reading material with a magnifying glass, or pay to have books enlarged by a publisher or copy shop, the long-term goal is never to be put off reading anything by the initial difficulty of small print. Making text larger is easy; developing an appetite for books, a hunger that will drive you to all necessary solutions, takes time.

PERIODICALS

There are many magazines and newsletters available in large print, some mainstream, some advocacy. Some are available through the NLS, and some have to be ordered directly from the publisher. You should call your NLS network library and request a copy of their catalog *Magazines in Special Media*, which profiles all specially formatted periodicals published by the NLS and other publishers and organizations.

AFB News. Newsletter chronicling activities of the American Foundation for the Blind, a leading organization in braille advocacy and publishing. Frequency: semiannual; cost: free; available formats: cassette, large print; publisher: American Foundation for the Blind, New York City, 800–232–5463.

Braille Book Review. Announces new braille books produced by the National Library Service, and updates on additional library services. Includes recorded version of *Talking Book Topics*. Frequency: bimonthly; cost: free; available formats: braille, electronic access, large print; publisher: The National Library Service. Request from regional library.

BVA Bulletin. Newsletter of the Blinded Veterans Association; it includes news on technology, legislation, employment, and association activities. Frequency: bimonthly; cost: free; available formats: cassette, large print; publisher: Blinded Veterans Association, Washington, DC, 800–669–7079.

Current Events. National school newspaper for junior high school students. Frequency: weekly; cost: est. $8.35 per year; available formats: braille, large print; publisher: American Printing House for the Blind, Louisville, KY, 800–223–1839.

Dialogue. Articles, poems, and stories by and about blind individuals; news; and columns on education, employment, sports, and daily living. Frequency: quarterly; cost: est. $28 per year; available formats: braille, cassette, computer disk, and large print; publisher: Blindskills, Inc., Salem, OR, 800–860–1224.

DVS Guide. Provides descriptions of upcoming PBS programs that use Descriptive Video Service; also includes news items on television's growing accessibility for the sight-impaired. Frequency: quarterly; cost: free; available formats: braille, cassette, large print; publisher: WGBH TV, Boston, 617–492–2777, ext. 3490, or 800–333–1203 (audio version).

New York Times Large Type Weekly. Weekly recap of national news, including business, people, features, sports, and reviews condensed from the *New York Times*. Includes cartoon and crossword puzzle in each issue. Frequency: weekly; cost: est. $70.20 per year; available formats, large print, flexible disk; publisher: New York Times Company, New York City, 800–631–2580.

Reader's Digest. Includes selections from the popular magazine anthology. Frequency: monthly; cost: est. $19.95 per year; available format: large print; publisher: Reader's Digest Fund for the Blind, Mount Morris, IL, 800–877–5293. Also publishes *Reader's Digest Large Type Reader*, which includes excerpts from condensed books, and *Great Biographies in Large Type*.

Tactic. Computer magazine for the sight-impaired, featuring the latest in adaptive technology and a readers' forum. Frequency: quarterly; cost: est. $25 per year; available formats: braille, computer diskette, large print; publisher: Clovernook Center, Cincinnati, OH, 513–522–3860.

Talking Book Topics. National Library Service publication listing all talking books recently added to the NLS collection. Frequency: bimonthly; cost: free; publisher, National Library Service. Request from regional library.

Tapping Technology. Comprehensive look at technological devices, services, and products to assist persons with disabilities. Frequency: monthly; cost: free; available formats: braille: cassette, computer diskette, large print; publisher: Tapping Technology, Baltimore, 800–832–4827.

Chapter 5: How to Find and Manage Readers

Being read to, as the cigar workers found out, allowed them to overlay the mechanical, mind-numbing activity of rolling the dark scented tobacco leaves with adventures to follow, ideas to consider, reflections to make theirs.

—Alberto Manguel, *A History of Reading*

THE NEED FOR READERS

There will be times when you need to read something unavailable in an alternative format and there is no time to have it transcribed, recorded, or enlarged. There will be times when you wish to read a magazine interview, CD lyrics, or the college newspaper. There are those moments when a teacher assigns a 20-page journal reprint to you for the following week's final. Moreover, you may sense moments when human interaction can enhance a reading in ways cassettes cannot—for instance, the pre-med student who reads your biology book to you, with endless offerings of easygoing elucidations.

For these reasons, the sight-impaired have much to gain by becoming adept at finding and working with readers, persons who will either read directly to you or will make tape recordings of material you select.

Developing relationships with readers is particularly important in college, where courses' required texts often are not known until the first day of class. And even if a book is available on tape, you may lose a week waiting for it to arrive. If the class is reading three books, and only two are available on tape or in braille, there may not be enough time for Recording for the Blind & Dyslexic or a braille transcription service to produce the book for you.

In addition to books, required reading might include articles, a professor's self-bound notes, and a chapter needed for a thesis—the cracks in special format publishing so easy to fall through.

Readers can get you through tough moments as a student, and open humane channels of interaction that can add many shades of meaning to new works you encounter.

WHERE TO FIND READERS

People love to read aloud. There is something about animating, reliving, or sharing a work through dramatic presentation that often makes it as exciting an activity for the reader as it is useful for the listener. And when the task is fused with a sight-impaired reader's genuine need for the service, the office becomes all the more attractive.

It is therefore easy to select and maintain a team of readers to whom you can assign different tasks to fill in any sudden gaps between what you need or wish to read, and the methods you normally employ.

Realizing that there are times when you need help and being able to ask for that help is not always easy. It may take time to feel comfortable reaching out. It should help you to know that reading to someone makes a person feel good, and it is one favor that is rarely refused.

Here are seven suggestions for finding readers.

1. Start in your home. Your mother or father—who read to you when you were a child—will often be glad to help you, and are the most understanding of your reading needs.

2. Tap your immediate circle: siblings, roommates, friends in your school classes or dorm, relatives, and friends of the family.

3. Ask your teachers, priest, minister, or rabbi, members of your church, or people recommended by your local librarian.

4. Have others find readers for you. Ask teachers if they know of anyone on the faculty or any students who might set aside time to read to you, or will make recordings.

5. Ask the local church to make an announcement at a weekly service or in the bulletin that readers are needed in the community, maintaining your privacy until volunteers step forward.

6. Call the local Lions Club (which provides services for the blind worldwide) and see if they can volunteer readers or donate extra tape recorders.

7. Put up a sign in your dorm elevator or local library. Free advertising of this kind can net you eager, competent readers.

Finding readers in college—the place where the sight-impaired often need them the most—is helped by the availability of reader's aid money from each state's department of education. A student is allotted a specific amount each semester to pay readers. The funds are usually sent to and administered by a liaison at the college's financial aid office, though the student is responsible for hiring readers, setting wages, and submitting monthly time sheets. Checks are mailed directly to the readers.

Classmates make great potential readers because they

have similar goals—they, like you, have to finish all the required reading in a course, and many will relish an opportunity to get paid at the same time.

Not that paying readers is a priority. Many, in fact, refuse payment, even from state funds their taxes help create. But late in the semester, when everyone is scrambling to prepare for finals, and you have 100 pages to plow through, finding a humanitarian to assist you gets a lot easier when you have $1,000 per year set aside.

WORKING WITH READERS

Whether people read to you out of the goodness of their hearts or to hear the sound of their own voice, you are neither a charity case nor a passive listener, and it is your responsibility to maintain a professional relationship. Whether or not you are paying them, you are a consumer of a crucial service that they have agreed to provide, and you have the right to have it done the way you want it.

Setting Goals

A professional relationship begins with your setting goals at the start of each period of crucial reading, whether that is a school year, a semester, or a time when you wish to read books for enjoyment.

Since reading yourself gives you more freedom and flexibility, your first step must be to consult the Louis Database on the American Printing House for the Blind website, or services such as Recording for the Blind & Dyslexic and the National Library Service, to determine if the book is available in an alternative format. At that time, you can also determine if having the book recorded or transcribed is an appropriate solution.

After you have a clear picture of what you need read, how soon you need it, and how long it will take, you will be able to determine how many readers you will need. Can the workload be handled by a single, dedicated reader, or does the need for help in several concurrent classes warrant spreading the work out over time and several readers?

Assessing Reader Interest

Knowing exactly what must be read up front will enable you to explain your precise needs to prospective readers, and will help readers immediately assess the degree to which they can help you achieve your goals.

For example, if you explain your situation to a roommate and ask if he can read to you from time to time, you have to make him understand right away that you are talking about two chapters of *Basic Meteorology* each week for a semester (which might work out to 32 one-hour sessions) and not an occasional letter from home.

Ask specific questions, such as "Can you read to me three hours per week for the semester for $4 per hour?" or "If I gave you a tape recorder and tapes, could you record the even chapters of this novel within the next two months?"

Be attentive and respectful to the usefulness of people's likes and dislikes. Your Stephen King-obsessed roommate might relish the opportunity to read those Edgar Allan Poe short stories for your American literature class. Your friend in the seminary might shy away from reading *Lady Chatterley's Lover*.

People find it hard to turn down a request to read, but

many view it as a singular act of community service, not something they prefer to do on a regular basis. Others will size up the reader's aid arrangement, and seek to install themselves as your Secretary of Reading.

Don't feel you must winnow out those who might be one-time readers. Take the hour or evening one friend graciously offers; there are other people who will be glad to help you on a more regular basis. Just remember that it is up to you to gauge the interest level of each individual.

The Reading Session

Another step in building a professional relationship is setting the time and place for each reading, being sure to arrive on time, and being respectfully attentive. In most cases, the reader is not being paid and thus is taking time out of his or her schedule to assist you. An appropriate response would be to accommodate the reader's preferences as to time and place.

Meeting at the reader's home, room, or office can make it easier for both of you. The reader will be able to work or relax right up to the time of the reading, and return to the day immediately after the session ends. He or she will also be more relaxed. You will benefit from being away from your usual surroundings, which might be relaxing and comfortable for you but can also detract from concentration on the material being read.

It is important to be alert and attentive while you listen. Although tape recorders and talking book machines allow your mind to wander and your head to droop, and even afford you the opportunity to do push-ups or clean your room while listening, an individual reader will see this as distracting and even disrespectful, like wandering up and down the aisles during a performance. The reader is providing the information you need, and deserves your undivided attention.

Taking notes, however, is usually not distracting, will help you get more from the session, and might prevent the need for a second reading.

Unless your reader enjoys long evenings under the lamp, try to keep sessions under an hour. That should get you through approximately 25 pages, and two or three such sessions per week should be enough to keep you caught up. If necessary, use a second reader between sessions.

Make it as easy as possible for people to read to you. Keep track of each book, and clearly mark the exact beginning and stopping points for each reading session. Give positive feedback on the previous session, reminding your reader what was covered, thus setting the stage for the current reading. Also, be prepared: bring extra paper, pens, and a dictionary to each session. Your reader might be curious about a word or allusion in a work, and might wish to jot down a note or do some underlining for you.

Giving Something Back

Readers usually ask for nothing, but your professional relationship with each one will be strengthened if you seek to give something back, to return the favor they have done for you. This something might be money, though reader's aid funds are available only for a brief period in one's life. A personal touch, an act that expresses your appreciation of a reader's time and assistance, may even be more valuable to a reader.

Give your reader breaks. Keep extra tape recorders and a supply of blank cassettes on hand, and offer readers a recording option. Some might prefer to help you that way.

If your reader is a classmate, you might record each session, listen to it again, and provide him or her with a written synopsis of what was read. This will help assure that you have grasped the material, and will be greatly appreciated by the reader. Words read aloud often are soon forgotten.

If a book or story touched you in a particular way, drop your reader a thank you note. Everyone wants to know their work is valued, and that happens all too infrequently.

You must discover and keep in mind what you like in the voice and delivery of prospective readers, and then act accordingly. The National Library Service, for example, indicates British-sounding narrators in its Mystery catalog. Such a choice is felicitous to some, pointless to others.

Chapter 6: Internet Resources

When the machine age has thus perfected its machines, it will be a means of life and not its despotic master. Democracy will come into its own, for democracy is a name for a life of free and enriching communion. We lie, as Emerson said, in the lap of an immense intelligence, but intelligence is dormant, and its communications are broken, inarticulate, and faint until it possesses the local community.

—John Dewey

This chapter describes some of the specific sites on the Internet that offer tools and information that can add new layers of access and efficiency to your reading. If you have a good idea of what the Internet is, and have used a computer at home or at school to access it, then you have already set foot on the next frontier of information delivery, and will be able to take advantage of new developments as they occur. If you are unfamiliar with the Internet, rouse yourself to learn; most of the crucial services described in this book are moving fundamental resources there.

The Internet is a worldwide interconnection of computer networks including sites maintained by companies, schools, organizations, and individuals that anyone can access through a computer that contains a modem and is connected to a standard telephone line. Sitting at a computer with Internet access and a web browser—a tool that allows you to access and display the contents of any page on any Internet site—you can quickly find and store information on virtually any subject that interests you.

It is the consumer portion of the Internet, the World Wide Web, that has exploded in popularity and general use in recent years, and it is the web and its many sites that most people mean when they refer to the Internet. When people speak of "surfing the web," they mean using their browser to access one site after another.

A site is a collection of information that a company, school, organization, or individual establishes (posts) and maintains; users access it via their browser. The amount of information contained on any site varies. It could be a four-line poem or a corporate repository of 10,000 separate documents.

A typical site for, say, an audiobook publisher might contain the company's complete catalog, a search engine to let you type in the title of a book to see if they have it, an order form, an electronic mail (E-mail) link for your instant correspondence, book excerpts that you can download and listen to, and links that, with one click, transport you to related sites.

In one on-line session, you might visit numerous sites, send E-mail messages to people all over the world, read any number of publications and print out articles, explore any hobby or interest, purchase items with a credit card, download free software and other useful information, get on mailing lists, enter chat rooms to meet people or share ideas, scan newsgroups and post messages, play games, check the weather, and a host of other tasks—some vital, some amusing, all with quick, unrestrained ease.

If you have a particular interest and want to see how

many sites are devoted to it, you can use what's called a search engine, such as Altavista, Lycos, or Yahoo. A search engine has a box where you enter key words (e.g., Star Trek, Etruscan pottery, Emily Dickinson) of the subjects you wish to explore. The engine quickly scans the entire World Wide Web and displays (usually in groups of 10 or 20) the sites whose descriptions best match your query. Some sites, like that of the hypothetical audio publisher mentioned above, might contain enough information to warrant having their own search engine.

It's easy to see what all the fuss is about—the web is an amazing development in our culture, affording the instant ability to regulate the flow of information into and out of our lives.

Of specific interest to sight-impaired readers, the Internet will further broaden the dynamic role of the personal computer as a reading tool. With its AudioPlus initiative, Recording for the Blind & Dyslexic is recording some textbooks in digital format that can be both listened to and read on the computer. As more and more books are converted to digital format, they will be available on CD-ROM, and later for download from the Internet. Eventually, a reader will be able to enter the RFB&D website, search the online catalog, select a book, download it onto a PC, and listen to it, using the computer's sound card and speakers. Other institutions, such as the National Library Service, are working with RFB&D to develop this technology.

Some sites already offer glimpses of future flexibility. One such site features electronic editions of many classics that can be copied to a computer's hard drive. The stored texts can later be read using a screen reader, or converted into a word-processing file for information searches, cutting and pasting, and other useful research paper and composition functions. Many audio publishers' sites offer clips that you can listen to. Others offer live readings, powerful search engines for locating hard-to-find books, and integrated catalog search and order functions that can dramatically shorten the time between being curious about a title and having read the book.

GETTING CONNECTED

If you do not own a personal computer, or are unfamiliar with the Internet, a quick way to get connected is to visit your school computer resource room or public library and ask for help in logging on. Once you know your way around, and are familiar with the terms and topography, you will see that the Internet is no more complicated to use than a telephone or TV set.

If you have a computer but are not currently using the Internet, you need to be sure your computer has a modem. Most recently manufactured computers were built with connectivity in mind and typically arrive with a modem already installed, and anything purchased for you by a state agency certainly will. If your computer does not have a modem, or if you wish to upgrade to one that is faster, it can be purchased and installed at a local computer store. The second requirement is connection to an outside phone line. This might be an additional phone jack on which you can share your home's current line, or a second line just for the Internet.

Depending on your level of vision, you may also need to have an internal speech synthesizer and screen-reading software installed on your system. A screen reader such as JAWS for Windows 3.2 will recognize and read any text on any web page. A description of adaptive technologies appears in Chapter 2.

After setting up the necessary hardware to make a connection, you need only install a browser or other software such as America Online (the software is free and often already installed on new computers), and follow the screen prompts to set up an account. These include the selection of a local access number that can be dialed for free from your telephone exchange (otherwise you will pay the long distance rate each time you log on), the selection and storing of an account or screen name and, in some cases, a password that gives you access to the service, and a method of payment (usually a credit card). A second phone line and an unlimited Internet account will cost between $50 and $75 per month.

Logging on requires a mere double click on the program icon, which dials and brings you to the home page of your chosen Internet service (American Online, CompuServe, or a local version maintained by an Internet service provider). A screen name and password are required; but many programs now let you store that information as a default that you activate with a press of the "Enter" key.

In most cases, the service's home page provides carefully arranged information on a variety of topics, such as links to late-breaking news stories, a place to check your E-mail, and easy access to an Internet search engine. America Online has a page of "channels" just behind the home page that puts users a click away from information on education, travel, games, shopping, personal finance, and the all-important Internet browser—your gateway to exploring and accessing individual sites all over the world.

To go to any site, such as the ones listed in this chapter,

merely type in its address in the Internet window or at the top of the page on the browser line and press "Enter." A web page address is as individual and pinpointed as a person's phone number, and once it is entered, your computer will call it up from whatever server it resides on and display it on your screen. You can move up and down each page, using the scroll bar, and from page to page within a site, or even jump to a totally new site by clicking on "hyperlinks" that appear either as underlined words or as indicative buttons or images. When the mouse pointer touches a hyperlink, its pointer image turns into a hand.

Another convenient navigation tool is a bookmark, a function that lets you store any page onto a list that you can instantly access from a drop-down menu at the top of the screen. Bookmarks are ideal for web pages you intend to visit frequently. The bookmark command is usually located on a menu at the top of the screen. Netscape Navigator calls them bookmarks and America Online calls them Favorite Places, but they work the same way. You might bookmark the home page of a service, like the American Printing House for the Blind, or a specific feature of that site, such as the Louis database. To access that page the next time you log on, simply click on the appropriate menu and select the stored page.

The remainder of this chapter suggests sites that you might bookmark as a way of beginning to use the web to enhance your efficiency and joy of reading by increasing your access to materials and services. The web changes so quickly that the information and sites you discover through browsing and surfing will give you the sort of up-to-the-minute expertise that cannot be found in books about the web or in most computer classes. The web is about information; being an active user on it lets you find, use, or ignore as much as you will ever need on any subject.

Clearinghouse Sites

Amazon.com	www.amazon.com
Audio Publishers Association	www.audiopub.org
Blind Net	www.blind.net/blindind.html
Braille on the Internet	www.nyise.org/braille.htm
Switchboard	www.switchboard.com
WebABLE	www.webable.com

Some sites make great points of departure, containing numerous links to other sites related to a topic, and thus giving you either a comprehensive road map, whose points you can jump to in an instant or, as with the on-line bookseller Amazon.com, a convenient hub of disparate materials. Among Amazon's 2.5 million titles are virtually all large-print, commercial audio, and disability titles from all major publishers and organizations. The Audio Publishers Association has links to over 100 websites that publish or resell books on cassette or CD-ROM (see selections below). BlindNet's two major links collections cover organizations related to blindness and companies specializing in adaptive products. Braille on the Internet covers all sites providing education and products, and braille history. WebABLE has over 200 links to sites dealing with all aspects of disability. Switchboard can help you search the web as well as find businesses and people by profession.

Foundation Resources Sites

American Foundation for the Blind	www.afb.org
American Printing House for the Blind	www.aph.org
National Association for Visually Handicapped	www.navh.org
National Federation of the Blind	www.nfb.org
National Library Service for the Blind & Physically Handicapped	lcweb.loc.gov/nls
Recording for the Blind & Dyslexic	www.rfbd.org

As noted in Chapter 1, the major blind services organizations maintain comprehensive websites. You should bookmark these immediately and visit them often, to stay up to date on technological advances, medical news, and opportunities such as scholarships and new publications. Three of the sites (APH, NLS, and RFB&D) contain catalogs that let you search more than 100,000 specially formatted books that will help you realize any school and personal reading goals. Most of these sites have audio clips you can listen to, either executive messages or recordings of ceremonies, as well as application procedures, catalogs and brochures that can be downloaded, and links to related sites focusing on education, technology, or daily living skills.

Audiobook Publisher Sites

Blackstone Audiobooks	www.blackstoneaudio.com
Broadcast.com	www.broadcast.com
HarperAudio/Caedmon	www.harperaudio.com
Listening Library	www.listeninglib.com
Recorded Books, Inc.	www.recordedbooks.com
Time Warner Audiobooks	pathfinder.com/twep/twab

These sites are included because they either sell unabridged books on tape (Blackstone Audiobooks, Listening Library, Recorded Books, Inc.) or provide classic works (HarperAudio/Caedmon) or have specialized study guides on cassette (Listening Library, Time Warner). Many sites (HarperAudio/Caedmon and Time Warner among them) also feature clips that you can download and listen to with a RealAudio player, a piece of software you can download at www.real.com. Broadcast.com is an especially dynamic future-pointing site, offering broadcasts of numerous radio programs, television programs, concerts, and a wide selection of audiobooks, all for free.

Education Sites

Easy Access to Software and Information	www.rit.edu/~easi
Internet Public Library	www.ipl.org
National Educational Association of Disabled Students	www.indie.ca/neads
Science—Engineering—Math (SEM)	www.asel.udel.edu/sem

Selected Social Studies Sites	www.cssjournal.com/sites.html
Teaching Math to Visually Impaired Students	www.tsbvi.edu/math

---

These sites offer subject-specific resources and access to a wide range of materials that can help sight-impaired students maximize learning effectiveness. EASI provides a wealth of information on educational technology, and holds on-line workshops on how to find and use adaptive computer aids. The Internet Public Library offers on-line access to numerous works of fiction, nonfiction, and references. The NEADS site, devoted to the empowerment of post-secondary students, has information on legislation, scholarships, and grants, and an on-line newsletter. The SEM site is funded by the National Science Foundation to encourage participation by disabled students in the fields of science, engineering, and math. The Selected Social Studies Sites are designed for teachers, but anyone can benefit from the links to sites covering history, archaeology, museums, maps, time lines, education, and the media. Math students can find information on the braille Nemeth code, including software translators and a free tutorial, tactile graphics, the abacus, talking calculators, and much more at the Teaching Math site.

ADDITIONAL SITES OF INTEREST

www.acb.org—The home page of the American Council of the Blind has much useful information on legislation, adaptive technology, and financial aid for the disabled.

www.assistivemedia.org—This site focusing on assistive media claims to be the net's first audioliterary service for persons with print reading/access barriers. The site's current offering is a David McCullough lecture on historical biography.

www.blind.state.ia.us/assist—The Iowa Department for the Blind offers free tutorials on using Windows and Windows applications with screen-reader software.

www.eblast.com—Eblast is a specialized search engine that lists the top websites on any given subject as chosen by the editors of the *Encyclopaedia Britannica*. Very useful on scholastic topics.

www.disabilityresources.org—A guide to hundreds of resources for all types of disability, including easy-to-use subject and geographical guides to top disability sites and services.

www.edc.org/FSC/NCIP—The National Center to Improve Practice seeks to promote the effective use of technology to enhance educational outcomes for students with sensory, cognitive, physical, and social/emotional disabilities.

www.nytimes.com—The *New York Times* web edition requires an application, but is free. The book review offers sample chapters and audio files that you can download.

www.poets.org—The site of the Academy of American Poets features text and audio samples from the country's greatest poets, as well as articles on related links.

www.research.att.com / cgi-bin / cgiwrap / mjm / voices.cgi— AT&T Bell Laboratories Voices page lets you play around with speech synthesis, allowing you to type in text and play it back in a variety of different voice styles.

www.rollingstone.com—The *Rolling Stone* Network contains not just the popular magazine but also radio programs, audio and video clips, and an archive where you can research your favorite musical performers.

www.viguide.com—This clearinghouse site on Internet resources on visual impairments is designed for parents and teachers. Links include special education, medical and legislative concerns, books, research, and entertainment.

zdnet.com—This site of computer trade journal publisher Ziff-Davis includes much useful information on computers, including product reviews, and has much to offer in the way of free downloads, tutorials, and on-line resources.

Chapter 7: Winning Strategies for Any Academic Reading Task

As mentioned earlier, the sole difference between sight-impaired readers and those with adequate vision is that the latter never have to think about how to go about reading, but simply read with their own eyes any material that is assigned or interests them. Those with sight impairments usually do not have such implicit freedom, but must develop a sense of what tools or organizations must be pulled in to complete any reading project. Doing this enough creates a sort of triage system for reading that can carry you through any task.

This chapter is designed to encourage you to think about developing such a system. We will look at some of the challenges one might face during a typical freshman year in high school. The techniques will work for any year or, for that matter, a summer of reading or a lifetime of continued learning with the use of books.

School is little more than chance meetings of your mind and new ideas and facts that teachers try and set up with their books, board work, reading assignments, and discussions. The goal is to touch off in your mind the sparks of recognition that will light you up the steps of knowledge.

But when one is blind, many lamps go unlit: long books are left unfinished; the images on the many maps, models, and mimeographs around the room cannot join the teacher's words to create that "aha" experience in the student's mind; the transparent ease of computer architecture cannot unlock a more linear conceptual level; and sight-impaired students usually cannot engage in sports and other will-defining activities.

If there is one ability that sight-impaired students must cultivate, it is keeping an inner eye on the future, and taking action to acquire all necessary materials. Preparing for ninth grade starts in eighth, with learning who next year's teachers are, perhaps introducing yourself at some point during the year, mentioning your disability, and letting that teacher know you will stop back in May to get a list of the books and other reading materials used in class. It's a process that takes little time, and plants positive images in people's mind.

Much of this work might be done for you (indeed, special education is designed to function this way), but there is nothing done that you cannot do better.

Once you know what agencies offer, and cultivate a habit of looking, you will hunt down and order books and other materials based on want as well as need—the way any consumer does—instead of taking what is given you.

Once you introduce yourself to new teachers and describe your disability in a forthright manner, you will receive more than assistance—you will have a chance to develop relationships that add efficiency and joy to schoolwork. Department meetings or memos flagging your entry into a new grade (the comment introduction) might leave some teachers not knowing what to expect or how to react. The initiative you take to let them know you as a person will make them eager to help.

ENGLISH AND READING

Benefits from a growing knowledge of how to order books from foundation resources such as the National Library Service and Recording for the Blind & Dyslexic will most immediately manifest themselves in classes such as English, where most literary works are available in a number of specialized formats. Most classics and many contemporary novels and anthologies are available in large print, on cassette or CD-ROM, and in braille. In some cases, you can obtain a work in more than one format, which might help you experience it on more than one level. A list of classic works culled from three separate book lists appears in Appendix C.

For this chapter, the sole point is to keep in mind the benefits of each of the various formats to ensure that you get the most from any given reading. For example, RFB&D has recordings of most classic novels, but narration quality is superior on NLS cassettes, whose production values are usually less than those of commercially produced books on tape. However, most commercial audiobooks are abridged, and NLS recordings state the page number (which might be important to cite on a paper) only at the beginning of each new track. Perhaps a combination of an NLS recording with a print copy of the book, or a second listening with an RFB&D recording, is the answer.

There are also large-print book providers such as the American Printing House for the Blind, and more affordable editions from commercial publishers.

Electronic texts, many of which can be downloaded for free from the Internet, offer still another way to read, listen to, or research a classic. New companies, such as Cyber Classics, sell editions of books in a double format: a crisp

14-point font print edition and a computer disk that can be used for research or read with a screen reader.

You have the right to choose which version or combination of versions suits your needs. You also have the responsibility to be sure these works end up in your hands. If you know that Stephen Crane's Civil War classic *The Red Badge of Courage* will be assigned next year, you can immediately call it in from RFB&D and the NLS (either in braille or on cassette), ask that the APH large type edition be ordered, borrow it from the NAVH library, or purchase it (abridged or unabridged) from any of 10 commercial publishers.

Such freedom might spur you on to locating materials and reading books long before they are assigned in class. Knowing what's coming will give you the time to have books brailled, enlarged, or recorded as need dictates.

Literary recordings in your high school and public library are another resource worthy of exploration, especially for dramatic works and poetry. You will no doubt have to read a few plays in high school, and productions by publishers such as Caedmon are the ultimate in literary listening. Their Shakespeare recordings, whose actors include Paul Scofield, Anthony Quayle, and Claire Bloom, may animate the language and give readers glimpses into Shakespeare's greatness better than any film or stage production can.

Developing relationships with librarians who might ease borrowing restrictions to accommodate your disability allows you to make recordings for one-time educational use, or even record works onto cassettes you provide, and can be a strong and lasting component of a lifelong reading program.

For those using reading systems or software, nearly 200

classics can be downloaded in their entirety for free on the Internet at the Alex Catalogue of Electronic Texts, located at http://sunsite.berkeley.edu/alex/. Cyber Classics (www. cybeclassics.com) sells paperback editions of many classics in crisp 12-point type. Each book comes with a 3 $\frac{1}{2}$-inch diskette that contains the complete text, which can be used for reading or writing.

MATH AND SCIENCE COURSES

Math and science are two subjects where recorded books are limited in their ability to replace the crucial connections between the eye or hand and the brain that result in learning. Whether it's with Nemeth braille, enlarged charts and diagrams, or tactile representations of geometric shapes, you have to encounter and manipulate much of the symbolism in math or science before you can grasp the concepts.

The American Printing House for the Blind has the most comprehensive selection of textbooks in braille and large print. In addition, they have many learning aids, such as the Geometry Tactile Graphics Kit, which teaches spatial concepts of lines and angles in a way some find superior to braille. For those with some residual vision, large-print texts are the ideal way to encounter math, where minute notations (exponents, angle degrees, etc.) are enlarged.

The same holds true for science. Tracking down and listening to a biology text is easy (RFB&D), but making arrangements, such as having books enlarged or brailled, finding useful products (like APH's new *Basic Tactile Anatomy Atlas*), or arranging for one-on-one guidance to learn dissection or lab help takes planning. Many braille transcribers cannot do Nemeth code; photos often lose clarity when enlarged; and listening to writing on chemistry or mathematics is not easy.

FOREIGN LANGUAGE CLASSES

Foreign language classes present a paradox for sight-impaired students. For the most part, all students enter beginning classes on the same level; there is much vocal participation (listening and repeating) that does not tax the eyes and, until advanced courses, there is little outside reading. Yet there are conjugation-lined placards, pronunciation charts with tiny accent marks over indecipherable letters, and a teacher writing tense constructions or participles across the blackboard.

With a little preparation, however, you can collect materials that can accelerate your progress and heighten your enjoyment of learning a new language. Such courses are, after all, one of the few areas of study with a rich tradition of learning through listening to recordings. As you develop your skills and a high comfort level with selecting and ordering tapes for other classes, tracking down vocabulary, conversation, or phonics tapes will be a smooth lateral step. A list of companies providing such materials is included below.

Another skill that is crucial to cultivate is being able to ask for one-on-one help, and perhaps budgeting time to meet with the teacher so that you can visually or tactilely absorb important concepts and distinctions that can escape the ears, such as letter or number variation, accent marks, grammar in action, and exact spellings. If the teacher holds up magazine ads in class as a vocabulary builder, make time to create your own large-type or braille flash cards. If the class watches a film or video, ask for a second screening where you can sit right in front of the monitor. Teachers are always happy to help when you take the initiative.

Some of the foundation resources provide specially formatted materials for learning a foreign language that can augment or amplify classroom work. Recording for the Blind & Dyslexic, for example, has many popular textbooks that, though produced by volunteer readers, possess a high quality of enunciation. The American Printing House for the Blind sells large-print workbooks and braille materials for learning 10 different languages, and produces many of the full-length works of literature distributed by the National Library Service (see Chapter 2).

Several commercial publishers specialize in foreign language materials, usually cassette or CD-ROM-based vocabulary programs. Some companies, including Audio Forum, also offer such things as word-a-day calendars, flash cards, software, and music.

Applause Learning Resources
85 Fernwood Lane
Roslyn, NY 11576
Phone: 516–365–1259
Toll free: 800–277–5287

Extensive selection of materials on popular languages (ESL, French, German, Italian, Japanese, Latin, Spanish, and Russian) for all levels of ability. Includes cassettes, software, magazines, maps, games, dictionaries, movies, and testing materials.

Audio Forum
96 Broad Street
Guilford, CT 06437

Phone: 203–453–9794
Toll free: 800–243–1234
Internet: http://agoralang.com/audioforum.html

Materials on nearly 100 different languages, from basic to advanced courses, to board games, song anthologies, and crossword puzzles.

Barrons Educational Series
250 Wireless Boulevard
Hauppauge, NY 11788
Toll free: 800–645–3476

Features Auto Language programs designed for those who already possess good general knowledge of a language, and Travel Wise courses, suitable for school language labs. Also has a wide variety of standardized testing preparation kits.

Berlitz International
400 Alexander Park
Princeton, NJ 08540
Phone: 609–514–9650
Toll free: 800–257–9449
Internet: www.berlitz.com

Berlitz has over 350 language centers worldwide, and for 120 years has sold an array of self-instructional language, reference, and travel materials. Included are basic and intermediate workbooks, picture dictionaries, phrase books, Think & Talk cassette programs, and business travel guides.

Heinle & Heinle
20 Park Plaza
Boston, MA 02116
Toll free: 800–354–9706
Internet: www.heinle.com

Comprehensive packages for learning French, German, Italian, and Spanish, as well as videos and professional development resources.

Penton Overseas
2470 Impala Drive
Carlsbad, CA 92008–7226
Phone: 760–431–0060
Toll free: 800–748–5804
Internet: www.pentonoverseas.com

A comprehensive audio publisher offering a wide range of cassettes on language, travel, and general education. Its VocabuLearn series features four cassettes teaching over 3,000 words (French or Spanish).

TESTING 101

As a blind student, you are entitled to special accommodations when taking standardized tests such as the Scholastic Aptitude Test (SAT), American College Testing Program (ACT), or subject-specific tests administered by your state, such as Regents' exams. You are entitled to a large-print or braille copy of the test, unlimited time to complete it, and, if you desire, a live reader to ask you the questions. The nature of such conditions might mean that a test like the SAT will be administered to you alone at your school, rather than the traditional mass testing held at various locations.

It is important to use all advantages to maximize scores. Though there may be better proof of one's sustained learning and intellectual suppleness than the SAT, the two-part test remains the one that every college relies upon. It is an exam that you can begin preparing for early in high school by concentrating on vocabulary and keeping up in math, and such vigilance can reinforce learning.

Unlimited time sounds like an unfair advantage to you, but will help only if your mind has stored the necessary information to begin with, and taking one's time can make for a long, tedious day of testing. The best way to prepare for the actual test is to take practice exams, and then to take the actual test more than once. Understanding how the test is scored is another key. Though some will counsel that a question left blank scores more favorably than an incorrect response, not answering questions limits your potential score. So learn all you can about the test, including how and when you can take it and whether you can take it online, and keep it in perspective as an opportunity to focus your acquisition of knowledge.

For more information on the standardized tests, contact the following:

American College Testing Program
Special Testing–61
ACT Universal Testing
2255 North Dubuque Road
PO Box 4028
Iowa City, IA 52243–4028
Phone: 319–337–1332
Internet: www.act.org

Corporate Headquarters
Educational Testing Service
Rosedale Road
Princeton, NJ
Phone: 609–921–9000
Internet: www.ets.org

The following books, all available through Recording for the Blind & Dyslexic, can provide additional assistance.

Cracking the SAT & PSAT
By Adam Robinson
New York: Random House, 1996
RFB&D shelf number: AB FF617

Gruber's Complete Preparation for the New SAT: Featuring Critical Thinking Skills, 7th ed.
By Gary R. Gruber
New York: HarperPerennial, 1996
RFB&D shelf number: AB FN269

SAT in a Week
By the Staff of the Stanley H. Kaplan Education Center
New York: Bantam Doubleday Dell, 1994
RFB&D shelf number: AB FK649

SAT, the Classic Course
By the Staff of the Stanley H. Kaplan Education Center
New York: Bantam Doubleday Dell, 1993
RFB&D shelf number: AB FQ397

Tooth and Nail: A Novel Approach to the New SAT
By Charles Harrington Elster
San Diego: Harcourt Brace & Co., 1994
RFB&D shelf number: AB FQ097

MUSIC-RELATED COURSES AND ACTIVITIES

Since 1962, the NLS has provided specially formatted materials to help blind and physically handicapped students deepen their knowledge of various aspects of music. Their extensive collection includes textbooks and musical scores in braille and large print, and elementary instructional cassettes for voice, piano, organ, guitar, recorder, accordion, banjo, and harmonica.

The best way to see if their collection contains items that

will be of use to you is to E-mail the Music Section at www.nlsm@loc.gov.

The organization's catalog *College Texts about Music* contains braille, cassette, and large-print books on a variety of music topics, including appreciation; history, literature, and criticism; harmony, theory, and ear training; form, style, and analysis; counterpoint; composition; orchestration and instrumentation; conducting ethnomusicology; acoustics; electronic music; reference; and textbooks designed for blind individuals.

In addition to its comprehensive catalog of musical scores in braille, the NLS maintains a list of certified music transcribers who will, for a fee, convert sheet music into braille. The names and addresses of these individuals can be found on the NLS website (www.loc.gov/nls/music/circular4.html).

PHYSICAL EDUCATION

The most important thing you will have to read here is the situation. To what degree you can involve yourself in gym classes and sports depends on many things, including which physical activities interest you and your level of vision. Total blindness may preclude participation in some sports or class activities, but there are few things that cannot be accomplished with a little planning to find or create the right situation. Blind athletes have excelled in such sports as swimming, judo, wrestling, cycling, and gymnastics, and have long participated in activities like bowling, golf, and hunting.

For those with a good deal of residual vision, opportunities to join team sports like cross-country and track open up. Yet these are often presented as alternatives to what others perceive as more visually preclusive sports like football and baseball. This is a decision only you can and should make.

As for gym classes, there may be health-related handouts that you have to wait to read until you can enlarge or scan the words, or exercise charts referred to in class that you might have to visit later or view with a monocular.

Other than that, you should take physical education very seriously, and ask for help in finding appropriate venues for participation, both from your gym teachers and from school administrators who might find necessary resources. One organization worth noting is the United States Association of Blind Athletes (USABA), located in Colorado Springs, which gets funding from the U.S. Olympic Committee, and which holds and provides scholarships for training camps in a number of sports. They can be reached at 719–630–0422 or on the web at www.usaba.org. Another great pace to start is Palaestra: The Forum of Sport, Physical Education, and Recreation for Those with Disabilities. They can be reached at 309–833–1902 or www.palaestra. com.

Appendix A: State-by-State Resource Guide

Many programs described in this book, such as the National Library Service, special education, and vocational rehabilitation, are federal mandates that are administered at the state level. It is therefore important to become well acquainted with the people who run these programs in your state.

The following guide lists the major reading-related service programs, institutions, and organizations in each state. These are not only there for you, but often because of you, and the tax dollars your family pays that fund the bulk of these programs. Call everyone. Tell them about yourself, your goals, your interests. Become the expert on what's going on in your state.

Since schools classify disabled students early on, special education and vocational rehabilitation departments will likely find you first. You should, however, develop your own idea of exactly what types of equipment and training you want from each of them. Special education should provide such things as additional tape recorders, all specially formatted books, and educational and testing materials, while vocational rehabilitation covers tuition, room and board, computer resources, and reader's aid. Never stop looking for devices or situations that might improve your education and reading life.

Getting to know your NLS librarian will help both of

you make better use of all available services. Contacting your state's National Federation of the Blind chapter to get their newsletter will ensure that you stay informed on legislative and social issues. This guide also lists additional state-specific reading services and organizations.

ALABAMA

NLS Regional and Subregional Libraries

Alabama Regional Library for the Blind and Physically Handicapped
6030 Monticello Drive
Montgomery, AL 36130
Phone: 334–213–3906
In-WATS: 800–392–5671
Fax: 334–213–3993
Internet: www.apls.state.al.us
Hours: 8:00–5:00, M–F

Department for the Blind & Physically Handicapped
Houston-Love Memorial Library
PO Box 1369
Dothan, AL 36302
Phone: 334–793–9767

Huntsville Subregional Library for the Blind & Physically Handicapped
PO Box 443
Huntsville, AL 35804
Bulk mail: 915 Monroe Street SW
Huntsville, AL 35801
Phone: 205–532–5980

Library and Resource Center for the Blind & Physically Handicapped

Alabama Institute for Deaf and Blind
705 South Street
PO Box 698
Talladega, AL 35160
Phone: 800–848–4722

Library for the Blind and Handicapped
Public Library of Anniston and Calhoun County
PO Box 308
Anniston, AL 36202
Phone: 205–237–8501

Tuscaloosa Subregional Library for the Blind & Physically
  Handicapped
Tuscaloosa Public Library
1801 River Road
Tuscaloosa, AL 35401
Phone: 205–345–3994

State Department of Special Education

Special Education Services Division
Department of Education
50 North Ripley Street
Montgomery, AL 36130–2001
Phone: 334–242–8114

Vocational Rehabilitation Services

Department of Rehabilitation Services
2129 East South Boulevard
Montgomery, AL 36116
Phone: 334–281–8780

National Federation of the Blind State Office

PO Box 963
Talladega, AL 35161
Phone: 205–937–3303

ALASKA

NLS Regional Library

Alaska State Library
Talking Book Center
344 West Third Avenue Suite 125
Anchorage, AK 99501
Phone: 907–269–6575
Fax: 907–269–6580
Internet: www.edu.state.ak.us/lam/library/dev/tbc.html
Hours: 8:00–4:30, M–F

State Department of Special Education

Office for Exceptional Children
Department of Education
801 West 10th Street Suite 200
Juneau, AK 99801–1894
Phone: 907–465–2970

Vocational Rehabilitation Services

Alaska Division of Vocational Rehabilitation
1016 West Sixth Street Suite 105
Anchorage, AK 99501
Phone: 907–274–5630

Center for Blind Adults
3903 Taft Drive
Anchorage, AK 99517
Phone: 907–248–7770

National Federation of the Blind State Office

3903 Taft Drive
Anchorage, AK 99517
Phone: 907–248–7770

ARIZONA

NLS Regional Library

Arizona State Braille and Talking Book Library
1030 North 32nd Street
Phoenix, AZ 85008
Phone: 602–255–5578
In-WATS: 800–255–5578
Fax: 602–255–4312
Internet: www.dlapr.lib.az.us
Hours: 8:00–5:00, M–F

State Department of Special Education

Superintendent of Public Instruction
Department of Education
1535 West Jefferson Street
Phoenix, AZ 85007
Phone: 602–542–4417

Vocational Rehabilitation Services

Rehabilitation Services Administration
Arizona Department of Economic Security
1789 West Jefferson Street, Suite 930A
Phoenix, AZ 85007
Phone: 602–542–6289

Arizona Center for the Blind and Visually Impaired
3100 East Roosevelt Street
Phoenix, AZ 85008
Phone: 602–273–7411

National Federation of the Blind State Office

2624 North Terrace Street
Mesa, AZ 85203–1225
Phone: 602–898–1188

ARKANSAS

NLS Regional and Subregional Libraries

Library for the Blind & Physically Handicapped
One Capitol Mall
Little Rock, AR 72201–1081
Phone: 501–682–1155
Fax: 501–682–1529
Hours: 8:00–5:00, M–F

Fort Smith Public Library for the Blind & Handicapped
61 South Eighth Street
Fort Smith, AR 72901
Phone: 501–783–0229

Library for the Blind and Handicapped
Northwest Ozarks Regional Library
217 East Dickson Street
Fayetteville, AR 72701
Phone: 501–442–6253

Library for the Blind & Handicapped, Southwest
CLOC Regional Library
PO Box 668
Magnolia, AR 71753
Phone: 501–234–1991

State Department of Special Education

Special Education Section
Department of Education
4 Capitol Mall
Education Building Room 105-C
Little Rock, AR 72201
Phone: 501–682–4221

Vocational Rehabilitation Services

Arkansas Division of Services for the Blind
522 Main Street Suite 100
Little Rock, AR 72201
Phone: 501–682–5463

National Federation of the Blind State Office

19 Brooklawn Drive
Little Rock, AR 72205–2304
Phone: 501–219–1680

Additional Resources

Lions World Services for the Blind
2811 Fair Park Boulevard
PO Box 4055
Little Rock, AR 72204
Phone: 501–664–7100

CALIFORNIA

NLS Regional and Subregional Libraries

Braille Institute Library Services
741 North Vermont Avenue
Los Angeles, CA 90029–3594
Phone: 213–663–1111, ext. 500
In-WATS: 800–808–2555
Fax: 213–663–0867
Hours: 8:30–5:00, M–F

Braille and Talking Book Library
California State Library
PO Box 942837
Sacramento, CA 94237–0001
Phone: 800–952–5666
Internet: library.ca.gov/california/State_Library/pubser/pubser
  05.html
Hours: 9:30–4:00, M–F

San Francisco Public Library
Library for the Blind and Print Handicapped
Civic Center
100 Larkin Street
San Francisco, CA 94102
Phone: 415–557–4253

Talking Book Library
Fresno County Public Library
Ted Wills Community Center
770 North San Pablo
Fresno, CA 93728–3640
Phone: 800–742–1011

State Department of Special Education

California Department of Education
Special Education Division
515 L Street Suite 270
Sacramento, CA 95814
Phone: 916–445–4613

Vocational Rehabilitation Services

Services for the Blind
Department of Rehabilitation
830 K Street Mall Room 208
Sacramento, CA 95814
Phone: 916–323–2235

National Federation of the Blind State Office

3934 Kern Court
Pleasanton, CA 94588–4428
Phone: 510–846–6086

Additional Resources

Beach Cities Braille Guild
PO Box 712

Huntington Beach, CA 92648
Phone: 714–969–7992

COLORADO

NLS Regional Library

Colorado Talking Book Library
180 Sheridan Boulevard
Denver, CO 80226–8097
Phone: 303–727–9277
In-WATS: 800–685–2136
Fax: 303–727–9281
Internet: www.cde.state.co.us/cdelib/ctbl.htm
Hours: 8:00–5:00, M–F

State Department of Special Education

Division of Special Education
Department of Education
201 East Colfax Avenue
Denver, CO 80203
Phone: 303–866–6694

Vocational Rehabilitation Services

Rehabilitation Field Services Division
Department of Human Services
110 16th Street Second Floor
Denver, CO 80203
Phone: 303–620–4156

National Federation of the Blind State Office

1608 Steele Street
Denver, CO 80206–1718
Phone: 303–321–4268

Additional Resources

Center for Independence
1600 Ute Avenue Suite 100
Grand Junction, CO 81501
Phone: 970–241–0315

CONNECTICUT

NLS Regional Library

Connecticut State Library
Library for the Blind & Physically Handicapped
198 West Street
Rocky Hill, CT 06067
Phone: 860–566–2151
In-WATS: 800–842–4516
Fax: 860–566–6669
Internet: www.cslnet.ctstateu.edu/lbph.html
Hours: 10:00–3:00, M–F

State Department of Special Education

Connecticut State Board of Education and Services for the Blind
170 Ridge Road
Wethersfield, CT 06109
Phone: 860–249–8525

Vocational Rehabilitation Services

Connecticut State Board of Education and Services for the Blind
170 Ridge Road
Wethersfield, CT 06109
Phone: 860–249–8525

National Federation of the Blind State Office

6 Cross Road Apartment 5
Stamford, CT 06905–3401
Phone: 860–289–1971

DELAWARE

NLS Regional Library

Delaware Division of Libraries
Library for the Blind & Physically Handicapped
43 South DuPont Highway
Dover, DE 19901
Phone: 302–739–4748
In-WATS: 800–282–8676
Fax: 302–739–6787
Hours: 8:00–4:30, M–F

State Department of Special Education

Director for Exceptional Children Team
Townsend Building
Federal & Duke of York Streets
Dover, DE 19903
Phone: 302–739–4601

Vocational Rehabilitation Services

Division for the Visually Impaired
Delaware Department of Health and Social Services
Herman Holloway Campus
1901 North DuPont Highway
Biggs Building
New Castle, DE 19720
Phone: 302–577–4731

National Federation of the Blind State Office

408 North James Street #13
Wilmington, DE 19804–3125
Phone: 302–999–7242

Additional Resources

Delaware Association for the Blind
800 West Street
Wilmington, DE 19801
Phone: 302–655–2111

DISTRICT OF COLUMBIA

NLS Regional Library

District of Columbia Regional Library for the Blind and Phys-
  ically Handicapped
901 G Street NW Room 215
Washington, DC 20001
Phone: 202–727–2142
Fax: 202–727–1129
Hours: 10:00–5:30, M–F

Department of Special Education

District of Columbia Special Education Branch
Goding School
920 Tenth Street NE
Washington, DC 20002
Phone: 202–724–4800

Vocational Rehabilitation Services

Rehabilitation Services Administration
Department of Human Services
800 Ninth Street SW Fourth Floor
Washington, DC 20024
Phone: 202–645–5807

National Federation of the Blind State Office

627 Dahlia Street NW
Washington, DC 20012–1841
Phone: 202–882–8090

Additional Resources

Columbia Lighthouse for the Blind
1421 P Street NW
Washington, DC 20005
Phone: 202–462–2900

The Metropolitan Washington Ear
25 University Boulevard East
Silver Spring, MD 20901
Phone: 301–681–6636
Internet: www.his.com/~washear

FLORIDA

NLS Regional and Subregional Libraries

Florida Bureau of Braille and Talking Book Library Services
420 Platt Street
Daytona Beach, FL 32114–2804
Phone: 904–239–6000
In-WATS: 800–226–6075
Fax: 904–239–6069
Hours: 8:00–5:00, M–F

Brevard County Library System
Talking Books Library
308 Forrest Avenue
Cocoa, FL 32922–7781
Phone: 407–633–1810

Broward County Talking Book Library
100 South Andrews Avenue
Ft. Lauderdale, FL 33301
Phone: 954–357–7555

Hillsborough County Talking Book Library
Tampa-Hillsborough County Public Library
900 Ashley Drive North
Tampa, FL 33602–3704
Phone: 813–273–3609 and 813–272–5727

Lee County Talking Books Library
13240 North Cleveland Avenue #54
North Fort Myers, FL 33903–4855
Phone: 941–995–2665

Orange County Library System
Audio-Visual Department
Talking Book Section

101 East Central Boulevard
Orlando, FL 32801
Phone: 407–425–4694, ext. 421

Pinellas Talking Book Library for the Blind and Physically
  Handicapped
12345 Starkey Road Suite L
Largo, FL 33773–2629
Phone: 813–538–9567

Talking Books
Palm Beach County Library Annex
7950 Central Industrial Drive Suite 104
Riviera Beach, FL 33404–9947
Phone: 561–845–4600

Talking Book Library
Jacksonville Public Libraries
1755 Edgewood Avenue West Suite 1
Jacksonville, FL 32208–7206
Phone: 904–765–5588

Talking Book Library of Dade and Monroe Counties
Miami-Dade Public Library System
150 NE 79th Street
Miami, FL 33138–4890
Phone: 305–751–8687

Talking Book Service
South Manatee Branch Library
6081 26th Street West
Bradenton, FL 34207
Phone: 941–742–5914

West Florida Regional Library
Subregional Talking Book Library
200 West Gregory Street

Pensacola, FL 32501
Phone: 904–435–1760

State Department of Special Education

Bureau of Instructional Support & Community Services
Department of Education
325 West Gaines Street Suite 614
Tallahassee, FL 32399–0400
Phone: 904–488–1570

Vocational Rehabilitation Services

Division of Blind Services
Florida Department of Labor
2551 Executive Center Circle
Tallahassee, FL 32399
Phone: 904–488–1330

National Federation of the Blind State Office

1949 Marseille Drive Apartment 2
Miami Beach, FL 33141–3455
Phone: 305–861–8425

GEORGIA

NLS Regional and Subregional Libraries

Library for the Blind & Physically Handicapped
1150 Murphy Avenue SW
Atlanta, GA 30310
Phone: 404–756–4619
In-WATS: 800–248–6701

Fax: 404–756–4618
Internet: www.gpls.public.lib.ga.us/LBPH.html
Hours: 8:00–5:00, M–F

Albany Library for the Blind and Handicapped
Dougherty County Public Library
300 Pine Avenue
Albany, GA 31761
Phone: 800–337–6251

Athens Talking Book Center
Athens-Clarke County Regional Library
2025 Baxter Street
Athens, GA 30606
Phone: 800–531–2063

Bambridge Subregional Library for the Blind & Physically
   Handicapped
Southwest Georgia Regional Library
301 South Monroe Street
Bambridge, GA 31717
Phone: 800–795–2680

Hall County Public Library
Library for the Blind & Physically Handicapped
127 North Main Street
Gainesville, GA 30505
Phone: 800–260–1598

LaFayette Subregional Library for the Blind & Physically
   Handicapped
305 South Duke Street
LaFayette, GA 30728
Phone: 706–638–2992

Macon Subregional Library
Physically Handicapped
Washington Memorial Library

1180 Washington Avenue
Macon, GA 31201–1790
Phone: 800–805–7613

Oconee Regional Library
Library for the Blind & Physically Handicapped
801 Bellevue Avenue
PO Box 100
Dublin, GA 31040
Phone: 800–453–5341

Rome Subregional Library for the Blind & Physically Handi-
capped
Sara Hightower Regional Library
205 Riverside Parkway NE
Rome, GA 30161–2911
Phone: 706–236–4618

Subregional Library for the Blind & Physically Handicapped
CEL Regional Library
2002 Bull Street
Savannah, GA 31499
Phone: 800–342–4455

Subregional Library for the Blind & Physically Handicapped
South Georgia Regional Library
300 Woodrow Wilson Drive
Valdosta, GA 31602–2592
Phone: 800–246–6515

Subregional Library for the Blind & Physically Handicapped
Talking Book Center
1120 Bradley Drive
Columbus, GA 31906–2800
Phone: 800–652–0782

Talking Book Center
Augusta-Richmond County Public Library

425 Ninth Street
Augusta, GA 30901
Phone: 706–821–2625

Talking Book Center
Brunswick-Glynn County Regional Library
208 Gloucester Street
Brunswick, GA 31523–0901
Phone: 912–267–1212

State Department of Special Education

Division for Exceptional Students
Department of Education
1870 Twin Towers East
Atlanta, GA 30334
Phone: 404–656–3963

Vocational Rehabilitation Services

Blind and Visually Impaired Program
Georgia Division of Rehabilitation Services
2 Peachtree Street 35th Floor
Atlanta, GA 30303
Phone: 404–657–3000

National Federation of the Blind State Office

390 Promenade Court SW
Marietta, GA 30064–3636
Phone: 770–590–7830

Additional Resources

Center for the Visually Impaired
763 Peachtree Street NE
Atlanta, GA 30308
Phone: 404–875–9011

GUAM

NLS Regional Library

Guam Public Library for the Blind and Physically Handicapped
Nieves M. Flores Memorial Library
254 Martyr Street
Agana, GU 96910
Phone: 671–472–6417 and 671–472–8264
Fax: 671–477–9777
Hours: 9:30–8:00, T & Th; 9:30–6:00, M, W, & F; 10:00–4:00,
  Sat; 12:00–4:00, Sun

State Department of Special Education

Department of Education
PO Box DE
Agana, GU 96932
Phone: 671–475–0562

Vocational Rehabilitation Services

Department of Vocational Rehabilitation
1313 Central Avenue
Tiyan, GU 96913
Phone: 671–475–4645

HAWAII

NLS Regional Library

Hawaii State Library
Library for the Blind and Physically Handicapped
402 Kapahulu Avenue
Honolulu, HI 96815
Phone: 808–733–8444
In-WATS: 800–559–4096
Fax: 808–733–8449
Hours: 9:30–4:30, M–Sat

State Department of Special Education

Special Education Section
Department of Education
3430 Leahi Avenue
Honolulu, HI 96815
Phone: 808–733–4999

Vocational Rehabilitation Services

Division of Vocational Rehabilitation
Hawaii Department of Human Services
Bishop Trust Building
1000 Bishop Street Room 615
Honolulu, HI 96813
Phone: 808–586–5366

National Federation of the Blind State Office

45–555 Poliahu Place
Kaneohe, HI 96744
Phone: 808–236–0690

IDAHO

NLS Regional Library

Idaho State Talking Book Library
325 West State Street
Boise, ID 83702
Phone: 208–334–2117
In-WATS: 800–233–4931
Fax: 208–334–2194
Internet: www.state.id.us/isuhp.htm
Hours: 9:00–5:00, M–F

State Department of Special Education

Special Education Supervisor
Department of Education
650 West State Street
Len B. Jordan Building Room 150
Boise, ID 83702
Phone: 208–332–6800

Vocational Rehabilitation Services

Idaho Commission for the Blind and Visually Impaired
341 West Washington
Boise, ID 83702
Phone: 208–334–3220

National Federation of the Blind State Office

1301 South Capitol Boulevard Suite C
Boise, ID 83706–2926
Phone: 208–343–1377

ILLINOIS

NLS Regional and Subregional Libraries

Illinois Regional Library for the Blind & Physically Handi-
  capped
1055 West Roosevelt Road
Chicago, IL 60608–1591
Phone: 312–746–9210
In-WATS: 800–331–2351
Fax: 312–746–9192
Hours: 9:00–5:00, M–F

Harold Washington Library Center
Talking Book Center
400 South State Street Room 5N7
Chicago, IL 60605
Phone: 800–757–4654

Mid-Illinois Talking Book Center Pekin Office
Alliance Library System
845 Brenkman Drive
Pekin, IL 61554
Phone: 800–426–0709

Mid-Illinois Talking Book Center Quincy Office
Alliance Library System
515 York
Quincy, IL 62301
Phone: 800–537–1274

Southern Illinois Talking Book Center
Shawnee Library System
607 Greenbriar Road
Carterville, IL 62918–1600
Phone: 800–455–2665

Talking Book Center of Northwest Illinois
PO Box 125
Coal Valley, IL 61240
Phone: 800–747–3137

Voices of Vision
Talking Book Center
DuPage Library System
127 South First Street
Geneva, IL 60134
Phone: 800–227–0625

State Department of Special Education

State Board of Education
100 North First Street, Room N-253
Springfield, IL 62777
Phone: 217–782–6601

Vocational Rehabilitation Services

Bureau of Blind Services
Illinois Department of Human Services
623 East Adams Street
PO Box 19429
Springfield, IL 62794–9429
Phone: 217–782–2093

National Federation of the Blind State Office

7020 North Tahoma Avenue
Chicago, IL 60646
Phone: 773–594–9977

Additional Resources

Chicago Lighthouse for People Who Are Blind or Visually Impaired
1850 West Roosevelt Road
Chicago, IL 60608
Phone: 312–666–1331

INDIANA

NLS Regional and Subregional Libraries

Indiana State Library
Special Services Division
140 North Senate Avenue
Indianapolis, IN 46204
Phone: 317–232–3684
In-WATS: 800–622–4970
Internet: www.statelib.lib.in.us/www.lbph/lbphO.html
Hours: 8:00–4:30, M–F

Bartholomew County Public Library
Fifth at Lafayette
Columbus, IN 47201
Phone: 812–379–1277

Blind and Physically Handicapped Services
Elkhart Public Library
300 South Second
Elkhart, IN 46516–3184
Phone: 219–522–2665, ext. 52

Northwest Indiana Subregional Library for the Blind and Physically Handicapped
Lake Country Public Library
1919 West 81st Avenue

Merrillville, IN 46410–5382
Phone: 219–769–3541, ext. 323 and 343

Talking Books Service
Evansville-Vanderburgh County Public Library
22 SE Fifth Street
Evansville, IN 47708–1694
Phone: 812–428–8235

State Department of Special Education

Department of Education
State House Room 229
Indianapolis, IN 46204
Phone: 317–232–4570
Fax: 317–232–4589

Vocational Rehabilitation Services

Blind and Visually Impaired Services
Indiana Family and Social Services Administration
Indiana Government Center
402 West Washington Street
PO Box 7083
Indianapolis, IN 46207–7083
Phone: 317–232–1433

National Federation of the Blind State Office

4017 Monaco Apartment B
Indianapolis, IN 46220
Phone: 317–466–7742

IOWA

NLS Regional Library

Library for the Blind and Physically Handicapped
Iowa Department for the Blind
524 Fourth Street
Des Moines, IA 50309–2364
Phone: 515–281–1333; 515–281–1389 (public access catalog)
In-WATS: 800–362–2587
Fax: 515–281–1378 and 515–281–1263
Hours: 8:00–5:00, M–F

State Department of Special Education

Bureau of Special Education
Grimes State Office Building
E. 14th & Grand Avenues
Des Moines, IA 50319
Phone: 515–281–4030

Vocational Rehabilitation Services

Iowa Department of the Blind
524 Fourth Street
Des Moines, IA 50309
Phone: 515–281–1333

National Federation of the Blind State Office

895 Fifth Avenue
Grinnell, IA 50112–1653
Phone: 515–236–3366

KANSAS

NLS Regional and Subregional Libraries

Kansas State Library
Kansas Talking Book Service
ESU Memorial Union
1200 Commercial
Emporia, KS 66801
Phone: 316–343–7124
In-WATS: 800–362–0699
Fax: 316–343–7124
Internet: skyways.lib.ks.uslkansas/KSL/talking/ksl_bph.html
Hours: 8:00–5:00, M–F

South Central Kansas Library System
Talking Book Subregional Library
901 North Main
Hutchinson, KS 67501
Phone: 800–234–0529, ext. 4

Talking Books
Northwest Kansas Library System
2 Washington Square
PO Box 446
Norton, KS 67654–0446
Phone: 800–432–2858

Talking Books
Topeka and Shawnee County Public Library
1515 SW 10th Avenue
Topeka, KS 66604
Phone: 800–432–2925

Talking Book Service
CKLS Headquarters
1409 Williams

Great Bend, KS 67530
Phone: 800–362–2642

Talking Book Service
Manhattan Public Library
North Central Kansas Libraries System
629 Poyntz Avenue
Manhattan, KS 66502–6086
Phone: 800–432–2796, ext. 152

Wichita Public Library
Talking Books Section
223 South Main
Wichita, KS 67202
Phone: 800–362–2869

State Department of Special Education

Student Support Services
Board of Education
120 Southeast 10th Street
Topeka, KS 66612–1182
Phone: 913–296–1413

Vocational Rehabilitation Services

Kansas Division of Services for the Blind
300 SW Oakley Biddle Building
Topeka, KS 66606–2807
Phone: 913–296–4454

National Federation of the Blind State Office

11905 Mohawk Lane
Shawnee Mission, KS 66209–1038
Phone: 913–339–9341

KENTUCKY

NLS Regional and Subregional Libraries

Kentucky Library for the Blind & Physically Handicapped
300 Coffee Tree Road
PO Box 818
Frankfort, KY 40602
Phone: 502–564–8300
In-WATS: 800–372–2968
Fax: 502–564–5773
Hours: 8:00–4:30, M–F

Northern Kentucky Talking Book Library
502 Scott Street
Covington, KY 41011
Phone: 606–491–7610

Talking Book Library
Louisville Free Public Library
301 York Street
Louisville, KY 40203
Phone: 502–574–1625

State Department of Special Education

Exceptional Children Service
Department of Education
Capital Plaza Tower Room 805
Frankfort, KY 40601
Phone: 502–564–4970

Vocational Rehabilitation Services

Kentucky Department for the Blind
PO Box 757

Frankfort, KY 40602
Phone: 502–564–4754

National Federation of the Blind State Office

3618 Dayton Avenue
Louisville, KY 40207–3736
Phone: 502–897–2632

Additional Resources

Audio Studio for the Reading Impaired
PO Box 23043
11403 Park Road
Anchorage, KY 40223
Phone: 502–245–5422

LOUISIANA

NLS Regional Library

Louisiana State Library
Section for the Blind & Physically Handicapped
760 North Fourth Street
Baton Rouge, LA 70802
Phone: 504–342–4943 and 504–342–4944
In-WATS: 800–543–4702
Fax: 504–342–3547
Hours: 8:00–4:30, M–F

State Department of Special Education

Louisiana Learning Resources System
State Department of Education

2758-C Brightside Lane
Baton Rouge, LA 70820–3507
Phone: 504–763–5431

Vocational Rehabilitation Services

Louisiana Rehabilitation Services
8225 Florida Boulevard
Baton Rouge, LA 70806
Phone: 504–925–4184

National Federation of the Blind State Office

2509 Foxx Creek Drive
Ruston, LA 71270–2512
Phone: 318–251–1511

Additional Resources

Lighthouse for the Blind in New Orleans
123 State Street
New Orleans, LA 70118
Phone: 504–899–4501

MAINE

NLS Regional Library

Library Services for the Blind & Physically Handicapped
Maine State Library
64 State House Station
Augusta, ME 04333–0064
Phone: 207–287–5650 and 207–947–8336

In-WATS: 800–452–8793 and 800–762–7106
Fax: 207–287–5624
Hours: 7:00–5:00, M–F

State Department of Special Education

Department of Education
23 State House Station
Augusta, ME 04333–0023
Phone: 207–287–5802

Vocational Rehabilitation Services

Division for the Blind and Visually Impaired
Maine Department of Labor
35 Anthony Avenue
State House Station #150
Augusta, ME 04333
Phone: 207–624–5323

National Federation of the Blind State Office

15 May Street
Portland, ME 04102–3710
Phone: 207–772–7305

Additional Resources

Maine Center for the Blind and Visually Impaired
189 Park Avenue
Portland, ME 04102
Phone: 207–774–6273

MARYLAND

NLS Regional and Subregional Libraries

Maryland State Library for the Blind & Physically Handicapped
415 Park Avenue
Baltimore, MD 21201–3603
Phone: 410–333–2668
In-WATS: 800–964–9209
Fax: 410–333–2095
Internet: www.sailor.lib.md.usilbphl
Hours: 8:00–5:00, M–F; 10:00–2:00, second Sat

Special Needs Library
Montgomery County Department of Public Libraries
6400 Democracy Boulevard
Bethesda, MD 20817
Phone: 301–897–2212

State Department of Special Education

Division of Special Education
State Department of Education
200 West Baltimore Street
Baltimore, MD 21201
Phone: 410–767–0238

Vocational Rehabilitation Services

Maryland Division of Vocational Rehabilitation Services
Administrative Offices
2301 Argonne Drive
Baltimore, MD 21218
Phone: 410–554–9405

National Federation of the Blind State Office

9736 Basket Ring Road
Columbia, MD 21045–3437
Phone: 410–992–9608

MASSACHUSETTS

NLS Regional and Subregional Libraries

Braille and Talking Book Library
Perkins School for the Blind
175 North Beacon Street
Watertown, MA 02172
Phone: 617–972–7240
In-WATS: 800–852–3133
Fax: 617–972–7363
Hours: 8:30–5:00, M–F

Talking Book Library
Worcester Public Library
3 Salem Square
Worcester, MA 01608–2074
Phone: 800–762–0085

State Department of Special Education

Massachusetts Department of Education
Educational Improvement Group
350 Main Street
Malden, MA 02148
Phone: 617–388–3300

Vocational Rehabilitation Services

Massachusetts State Commission for the Blind
88 Kingston Street
Boston, MA 02111
Phone: 617–727–5550, ext. 4503

National Federation of the Blind State Office

55 Delaware Avenue
Somerset, MA 02726–3714
Phone: 508–679–8543

Additional Resources

Massachusetts Association for the Blind
200 Ivy Street
Brookline, MA 02146
Phone: 617–738–5110
Toll free (in Massachusetts): 800–682–9200

Carroll Center for the Blind
770 Centre Street
Newton, MA 02158–2597
Phone: 617–969–6200
Toll free (in Massachusetts): 800–852–3131

MICHIGAN

NLS Regional and Subregional Libraries

Library of Michigan
Service for the Blind and Physically Handicapped
PO Box 30007
Lansing, MI 48909

Phone: 517–373–5614
In-WATS: 800–992–9012
Fax: 517–373–5865
Internet: www.libofmich.lib.mi.uslcitizens/collections/
  sbphbrochure.html
Hours: 8:00–5:00, M–F

Downtown Detroit Subregional Library for the Blind & Physically Handicapped
121 Gratiot Avenue
Detroit, MI 48226
Phone: 313–224–0580

Grand Traverse Area Library for the Blind & Physically Handicapped
322 Sixth Street
Traverse City, MI 49684
Phone: 616–922–4824

Kent District Library for the Blind and Physically Handicapped
775 Ball Avenue NE
Grand Rapids, MI 49503–1307
Phone: 616–336–3262

Macomb Library for the Blind & Physically Handicapped
16480 Hall Road
Clinton Township, MI 48038–1132
Phone: 810–286–1580

Muskegon County Library for the Blind & Physically Handicapped
635 Ottawa Street
Muskegon, MI 49442
Phone: 616–724–6257

Northland Library Cooperative
316 East Chisholm Street

Alpena, MI 49707
Phone: 800–446–1580

Oakland County Library for the Blind & Physically Handi-
   capped
1200 North Telegraph Department 482
Pontiac, MI 48341–0482
Phone: 810–858–5050
In-WATS: 800–774–4542 (Oakland County)

St. Clair County Library for the Blind & Physically Handicapped
210 McMorran Boulevard
Port Huron, MI 48060
Phone: 800–272–8570

Talking Book Center
Mideastern Michigan Library for the Blind & Physically Handi-
   capped
G-4195 West Pasadena Avenue
Flint, MI 48504
Phone: 810–732–1120

Upper Peninsula Library for the Blind & Physically Handicapped
1615 Presque Isle Avenue
Marquette, MI 49855
Phone: 800–562–8985

Washtenaw County Library for the Blind & Physically Handi-
   capped
PO Box 8645
Ann Arbor, MI 48107–8645
Phone: 313–971–6059

Wayne County Regional Library for the Blind & Physically
   Handicapped
33030 Van Born Road

Wayne, MI 48184
Phone: 313–274–2600

State Department of Special Education

Office of Special Education
Department of Education
PO Box 30008
Lansing, MI 48909
Phone: 517–373–9433

Vocational Rehabilitation Services

Commission for the Blind
Family Independence Agency
201 North Washington Square
PO Box 30652
Lansing, MI 48909
Phone: 517–373–2062

National Federation of the Blind State Office

15688 Woodland Drive
Dearborn, MI 48120–1112
Phone: 313–271–8700

Additional Resources

Association for the Blind & Visually Impaired
215 Sheldon SE
Grand Rapids, MI 49503
Phone: 616–458–1187

Newspapers for the Blind
PO Box 441

Clio, MI 48420
Phone: 810–762–3656

MINNESOTA

NLS Regional Library

Minnesota Library for the Blind & Physically Handicapped
P.O. Box 68 Highway 298
Faribault, MN 55021
Phone: 507–332–3279
Fax: 507–332–3260
Hours: 7:30–5:00, M–F

State Department of Special Education

Division of Special Education
Department of Children, Families & Learning
550 Cedar Street, Seventh Floor
St. Paul, MN 55101
Phone: 612–296–1793

Vocational Rehabilitation Services

Minnesota State Services for the Blind and Visually Handi-
    capped
2200 University Avenue West Suite 240
St. Paul, MN 55114
Phone: 612–642–0500

National Federation of the Blind State Office

5132 Queen Avenue South
Minneapolis, MN 55410–2217
Phone: 612–920–0959

Additional Resources

Lighthouse for the Blind
4505 West Superior Street
Duluth, MN 55807
Phone: 218–624–4828

MISSISSIPPI

NLS Regional Library

Mississippi Library Commission
Talking Book and Braille Services
5455 Executive Place
Jackson, MS 39206
Phone: 601–354–7208
In-WATS: 800–446–0892
Fax: 601–354–6077
Internet: www.mlc.state.ms.us/tbbs.htm
Hours: 7:30–5:00, M–F

State Department of Special Education

Bureau of Special Education
Department of Education
PO Box 771
Jackson, MS 39205
Phone: 601–359–3513

Vocational Rehabilitation Services

Office of Vocational Rehabilitation for the Blind
Mississippi Department of Rehabilitation Services
PO Box 1698

Jackson, MS 39215–1698
Phone: 601–853–5100

National Federation of the Blind State Office

268 Lexington Avenue
Jackson, MS 39209–5431
Phone: 601–355–1054

MISSOURI

NLS Regional Library

Wolfner Library for the Blind & Physically Handicapped
PO Box 387
Jefferson City, MO 65102–0387
Phone: 573–751–8720
In-WATS: 800–392–2614
Fax: 573–526–2985
Internet:mosl/sos.state.mo.us/libser/wolf/wolf.html
Hours 8:00–5:00, M–F

State Department of Education

Division of Special Education
Department of Elementary & Secondary Education
Jefferson Building Sixth Floor
PO Box 480
Jefferson City, MO 65102
Phone: 573–751–4909

Vocational Rehabilitation Services

Missouri Rehabilitation Services for the Blind
3418 Knipp Drive
Jefferson City, MO 65109
Phone: 573–751–4249

National Federation of the Blind State Office

1209 Ireland Court
Columbia, MO 65203–2088
Phone: 573–874–1774

Additional Resources

Alphapointe Association for the Blind
1844 Broadway
Kansas City, MO 64108
Phone: 816–421–5848

MONTANA

NLS Regional Library

Montana Talking Book Library
1515 East Sixth Avenue
Helena, MT 59620
Phone: 406–444–2064
In-WATS: 800–332–3400
Fax: 406–444–5612
Hours: 8:00–5:00, M–F

State Department of Special Education

Division of Special Education
Montana Department of Curriculum
Capitol Station
Helena, MT 59620
Phone: 406–444–4429

Vocational Rehabilitation Services

Disability Services Division
Department of Public Health & Human Services
111 Sanders Street
Helena, MT 59620
Phone: 406–444–2590

National Federation of the Blind State Office

2724 Amherst Avenue
Butte, MT 59701–4239
Phone: 406–494–4571

NEBRASKA

NLS Regional Library

Nebraska Library Commission
Talking Book and Braille Service
The Atrium
1200 N Street Suite 120
Lincoln, NE 68508–2023
Phone: 402–471–4038
In-WATS: 800–742–7691
Fax: 402–471–6244

Internet: www.nlc.state.ne.us/tbbs/tbbsl.html
Hours: 8:00–5:00, M–F

State Department of Special Education

Special Education Branch
Department of Education
PO Box 94987
Lincoln, NE 68509
Phone: 402–471–2471

Vocational Rehabilitation Services

Nebraska Division of Rehabilitation
Services for the Visually Impaired
4600 Valley Road
Lincoln, NE 68510–4844
Phone: 402–471–2891

National Federation of the Blind State Office

868 South 44th Street
Lincoln, NE 68510–4705
Phone: 402–488–4245

NEVADA

NLS Regional and Subregional Libraries

Nevada State Library and Archives
Regional Library for the Blind & Physically Handicapped
Capitol Complex
Carson City, NV 89701
Phone: 702–687–5154

In-WATS: 800–922–9334
Fax: 702–687–8311
Internet: www.clan.lib.nv.us/docs/tbooks.htm
Hours: 8:00–5:00, M–F

Subregional Library for the Blind & Handicapped
Las Vegas-Clark County Library District
1401 East Flamingo Road
Las Vegas, NV 89119
Phone: 702–733–1925

State Department of Special Education

Special Education
Department of Education
700 East Fifth Street
Carson City, NV 89701
Phone: 702–687–9123

Vocational Rehabilitation Services

Nevada Bureau of Services to the Blind
Department of Human Resources
505 East King Street
Carson City, NV 89710
Phone: 702–687–4440

National Federation of the Blind State Office

6817 Beach Nest Avenue
Las Vegas, NV 89130–1774
Phone: 702–396–5515

NEW HAMPSHIRE

NLS Regional Library

New Hampshire State Library
Library Services to Persons with Disabilities
117 Pleasant Street
Concord, NH 03301–3852
Phone: 603–271–3429
In-WATS: 800–491–4200
Fax: 603–226–2907 Sept–May or 603–271–6826 June–Aug
Internet: www.state.nh.us/nhsl/talking.html
Hours: 8:00–4:30, M–F

State Department of Special Education

Educational Improvement Division
New Hampshire Department of Education
101 Pleasant Street
Concord, NH 03301–3890
Phone: 603–271–6051

Vocational Rehabilitation Services

Services to the Blind and Visually Handicapped
New Hampshire Division of Vocational Rehabilitation
78 Regional Drive Building 2
Concord, NH 03301–8508
Phone: 603–271–3537

National Federation of the Blind State Office

2 Center Street Apartment 1
Laconia, NH 03246–3737
Phone: 603–524–7164

Additional Resources

New Hampshire Association for the Blind
25 Walker Street
Concord, NH 03301
Phone: 603–224–4039
Toll free (in New Hampshire): 800–464–3075

NEW JERSEY

NLS Regional Library

New Jersey Library for the Blind & Handicapped
2300 Stuyvesant Avenue CN 501
Trenton, NJ 08625–0501
Phone: 609–292–6450
In-WATS: 800–792–8322 (English) or 800–582–5945 (Spanish)
Fax: 609–530–6384
Internet: www.state.nj.us/statelibrary/njlbh.htm
Hours: 9:00–4:30, M–F; 9:00–3:00, Sat

State Department of Special Education

Office of Special Education
Department of Education
100 Riverview Plaza Second Floor
CN 500
Trenton, NJ 08625
Phone: 609–292–0147

Vocational Rehabilitation Services

Commission for the Blind and Visually Impaired
153 Halsey Street

PO Box 47017
Newark, NJ 07101
Phone: 201–648–2324

National Federation of the Blind State Office

69 Prospect Place
Belleville, NJ 07109–2526
Phone: 201–759–3622

NEW MEXICO

NLS Regional Library

New Mexico State Library
Talking Book Library
325 Don Gaspar
Santa Fe, NM 87501–2777
Phone: 505–827–3830
In-WATS: 800–456–5515
Fax: 505–827–3888
Internet: www.sflib.state.nm.us/tbl.prog-info/tblpage.html
Hours: 9:00–5:00, M–F

State Department of Special Education

Special Education Office
Department of Education
Education Building
300 Don Gaspar Street
Santa Fe, NM 87501
Phone: 505–827–6541

Vocational Rehabilitation Services

New Mexico Commission for the Blind
PERA Building Room 553
Santa Fe, NM 87503
Phone: 505–827–4479

National Federation of the Blind State Office

PO Box 7900
Albuquerque, NM 87194
Phone: 505–243–6165

Additional Resources

Newsline for the Blind
New Mexico Commission for the Blind
2200 Yale Boulevard Southeast
Albuquerque, NM 87106
Phone: 505–841–8844

NEW YORK

NLS Regional Libraries

Long Island

Talking Books Plus
Outreach Services
Suffolk Cooperative Library System
627 North Sunrise Service Road
Bellport, NY 11713
Phone: 516–286–1600

Talking Books
Nassau Library System
900 Jerusalem Avenue
Uniondale, NY 11553
Phone: 516–292–8920

New York City

Andrew Heiskell Library for the Blind & Physically Handi-
    capped
New York Public Library
40 West 20th Street
New York, NY 10011–4211
Phone: 212–206–5400

Upstate

New York State Talking Book and Braille Library
Cultural Education Center
Empire State Plaza
Albany, NY 12230
Phone: 518–474–5935
In-WATS: 800–342–3688
Fax: 518–474–5786
Internet: www.nysl.nysed.gov/talk.htm
Hours: 8:00–4:30, M–F

State Department of Special Education

New York State Education Department
Office for Special Education Services
One Commerce Plaza Room 1624
Albany, NY 12234
Phone: 518–486–9592

Vocational Rehabilitation Services

New York State Commission for the Blind and Visually Handicapped
40 North Pearl Street
Albany, NY 12243
Phone: 518–473–1801

National Federation of the Blind State Office

471 63rd Street
Brooklyn, NY 11220–4617
Phone: 718–492–5871

Additional Resources

The Lighthouse Inc.
111 East 59th Street
New York, NY 10022–1202
Phone: 212–821–9200
Toll free: 800–334–5497
Internet: www.lighthouse.org

Jewish Guild for the Blind
15 West 65th Street
New York, NY 10023
Phone: 212–769–6200

NORTH CAROLINA

NLS Regional Library

North Carolina Library for the Blind & Physically Handicapped
State Library of North Carolina
Department of Cultural Resources

1811 Capital Boulevard
Raleigh, NC 27635
Phone: 919–733–4376
In-WATS: 800–662–7726
Fax: 919–733–6910
Internet: www.dcr.state.nc.us/about.htm#lbph
Hours: 8:00–5:00, M–F

State Department of Special Education

Exceptional Children Division
Department of Public Instruction
301 North Wilmington Street
Raleigh, NC 27601–2825
Phone: 919–715–1565

Vocational Rehabilitation Services

Department of Human Resources
Division of Services for the Blind
309 Ashe Avenue
Raleigh, NC 27606
Phone: 919–733–9700

National Federation of the Blind State Office

1205 Snowhill Road
Durham, NC 27712
Phone: 919–477–0445

NORTH DAKOTA

NLS Regional Library

North Dakota State Library
Talking Book Services

604 East Boulevard
Bismarck, ND 58505–0800
Phone: 701–328–1477
In-WATS: 800–843–9948
Fax: 701–328–2040
Internet: www.sendit.nodak.edu/ndsl/hand/html
Hours: 8:00–5:00, M–F

State Department of Special Education

Special Education
Department of Public Instruction
State Capitol 10th Floor
600 East Boulevard Avenue
Bismarck, ND 58505–0440
Phone: 701–328–2277

Vocational Rehabilitation Services

Vocational Rehabilitation
North Dakota Department of Human Services
600 South Second Street
Dacotah Foundation Building
Bismarck, ND 58504
Phone: 701–328–8950

National Federation of the Blind State Office

4445 Santiago Boulevard
Fargo, ND 58103–1069
Phone: 701–281–1374

OHIO

NLS Regional and Subregional Libraries

Public Library of Cincinnati & Hamilton County
Library for the Blind & Physically Handicapped
800 Vine Street Library Square
Cincinnati, OH 45202–2071
Phone: 513–369–6999
In-WATS: 800–582–0335
Fax: 513–369–3111
Internet: plch.lib.oh.us/plch/main/43.htm
Hours: 8:00–9:00, M–F; 9:00–6:00, Sat; 1:00–5:00, Sun

Northern Ohio

Library for the Blind & Physically Handicapped
Cleveland Public Library
17121 Lake Shore Boulevard
Cleveland, OH 44110–4006
Phone: 216–623–2911
In-WATS: 800–362–1262

State Department of Special Education

Division of Special Education
Department of Education
933 High Street
Worthington, OH 43085
Phone: 614–466–2650

Vocational Rehabilitation Services

Rehabilitation Services Commission
400 East Campus View Boulevard

Columbus, OH 43235
Phone: 614–438–1255

National Federation of the Blind State Office

237 Oak Street
Oberlin, OH 44074–1517
Phone: 800–396–6326

OKLAHOMA

NLS Regional Library

Oklahoma Library for the Blind & Physically Handicapped
300 NE 18th Street
Oklahoma City, OK 73105
Phone: 405–521–3514
In-WATS: 800–523–0288
Fax: 405–521–4582
Hours: 8:00–5:00, M–F

State Department of Special Education

Special Education Section
Department of Education
2500 North Lincoln Boulevard
Oklahoma City, OK 73005
Phone: 405–521–3351

Vocational Rehabilitation Services

State Department of Rehabilitation
Visual Services Division
3535 Northwest 58th Street Suite 500

Oklahoma City, OK 73112
Phone: 405–951–3400

National Federation of the Blind State Office

101 North Easy Street
Edmond, OK 73105
Phone: 405–629–6550

Additional Resources

Oklahoma League for the Blind
PO Box 24020
Oklahoma City, OK 73124
Phone: 405–232–4644

OREGON

NLS Regional Library

Oregon State Library
Talking Book and Braille Services
250 Winter Street NE
Salem, OR 97310–0645
Phone: 503–378–3849 and 503–224–0610
Toll free in Oregon: 800–452–0292 (except Portland)
Fax: 503–588–7119
Internet: www.osl.state.onus/tbabs/tbabs.html
Hours: 8:00–5:00, M–F

State Department of Special Education

Office of Special Education
Division of Special Student Services

Department of Education
255 Capitol Street SE
Salem, OR 97310
Phone: 503–378–3598

Vocational Rehabilitation Services

Oregon Commission for the Blind
535 SE 12th Avenue
Portland, OR 97214
Phone: 503–731–3221

National Federation of the Blind State Office

PO Box 320
Thurston, OR 97482
Phone: 541–726–6924

PENNSYLVANIA

NLS Regional Libraries

East

Library for the Blind & Physically Handicapped
Free Library of Philadelphia
919 Walnut Street
Philadelphia, PA 19107
Phone: 215–925–3213
In-WATS: 800–222–1754
Fax: 215–928–0856
Internet: libertynet.org/~asbinfo/library.html
Hours: 9:00–5:00, M–F

West

Library for the Blind & Physically Handicapped
Carnegie Library of Pittsburgh
Leonard C. Staisey Building
4724 Baum Boulevard
Pittsburgh, PA 15213–1389
Phone: 412–687–2440
In-WATS: 800–242–0586
Fax: 412–687–2442
Internet: www.clgph.org/CLP/LBPH/intro.html
Hours: 9:00–5:00, M–F

State Department of Special Education

Bureau of Special Education
Department of Education
333 Market Street Seventh Floor
Harrisburg, PA 17126
Phone: 717–783–6913

Vocational Rehabilitation Services

Bureau of Blindness and Visual Services
Pennsylvania Department of Public Welfare
1401 North Seventh Street
PO Box 2675
Harrisburg, PA 17105
Phone: 717–787–6176
Toll free (in Pennsylvania): 800–622–2842

National Federation of the Blind State Office

42 South 15th Street
Robinson Building Suite 320

Philadelphia, PA 18102–2203
Phone: 215–988–0888

Additional Resources

Associated Services for the Blind
919 Walnut Street
Philadelphia, PA 19107
Phone: 215–627–0600

York County Blind Center
1380 Spahn Avenue
York, PA 17403
Phone: 717–848–1690

PUERTO RICO

NLS Regional Library

Puerto Rico Regional Library for the Blind & Physically Handi-
    capped
520 Ponce de Leon Avenue
San Juan, PR 00901
Phone: 787–723–2519
In-WATS: 800–981–8008
Fax: 787–721–8177
Hours: 7:30–5:00, M–F

Department of Special Education

Special Education Section
Department of Education
PO Box 759
Hato Rey, PR 00919
Phone: 787–759–2000

Vocational Rehabilitation Services

Vocational Rehabilitation Program
Puerto Rico Department of Social Services
PO Box 191118
San Juan, PR 00919–1118
Phone: 787–724–3120

RHODE ISLAND

NLS Regional Library

Talking Books Plus: Rhode Island Regional Library for the
  Blind & Physically Handicapped
Office of Library and Information Services
One Capitol Hill
Providence, RI 02908
Phone: 401–277–2726
In-WATS: 800–734–5141
Fax: 401–277–4195
Internet: www.doa.state.ri.us/dsls/dept/lbphhome.htm
Hours: 8:30–4:00, M–F

State Department of Special Education

Office of Special Needs
Department of Education
22 Hayes Street
Providence, RI 02903
Phone: 401–277–3505

Vocational Rehabilitation Services

Services for the Blind and Visually Impaired
40 Fountain Street
Providence, RI 02903
Phone: 401–277–2300

National Federation of the Blind State Office

324 Dover Avenue
East Providence, RI 02914–3145
Phone: 401–433–2606

Additional Resources

IN-SIGHT: Rhode Island Association for the Blind
43 Jefferson Boulevard
Warwick, RI 02888
Phone: 401–941–3322

SOUTH CAROLINA

NLS Regional Library

South Carolina State Library
Department for the Blind & Physically Handicapped
301 Gervais Street
PO Box 821
Columbia, SC 29202–0821
Phone: 803–737–9970
In-WATS: 800–922–7818
Fax: 803–737–9983
Internet: www.state.sc.us/scsl/talkbook.html
Hours: 8:30–5:00, M–F

State Department of Special Education

Office of Programs for Exceptional Children
South Carolina Department of Education
Rutledge Office Building
1429 Senate Street
Columbia, SC 29201
Phone: 803–734–8222

Vocational Rehabilitation Services

South Carolina Commission for the Blind
1430 Confederate Avenue
Columbia, SC 29201
Phone: 803–734–7520
Toll free (in South Carolina): 800–922–2222

National Federation of the Blind State Office

1829 Belmont Drive
Columbia, SC 29206–2813
Phone: 803–787–0462

Additional Resources

Association for the Blind
2209 Mechanic Street
Charleston, SC 29405
Phone: 803–723–6915

SOUTH DAKOTA

NLS Regional Library

South Dakota Braille and Talking Book Library
State Library Building

800 Governors Drive
Pierre, SD 57501–2294
Phone: 605–773–3514
In-WATS: 800–423–6665
Fax: 605–773–4950
Internet: state.sd.us/state/executive/deca/st_lib/talkbook/
Hours: 8:00–5:00, M–F

State Department of Special Education

Office of Special Education
Division of Education
700 Governors Drive
Pierre, SD 57501
Phone: 605–773–3678

Vocational Rehabilitation Services

Division of Services to the Blind and Visually Impaired
Department of Human Services
Hillsview Plaza
500 East Capitol Avenue
Pierre, SD 57501
Phone: 605–773–4644

National Federation of the Blind State Office

919 Main Street Suite 15
Rapid City, SD 57701–2662
Phone: 605–342–3885

TENNESSEE

NLS Regional Library

Tennessee Library for the Blind & Physically Handicapped
Tennessee State Library and Archives
403 Seventh Avenue North
Nashville, TN 37243–0313
Phone: 615–741–3915
In-WATS: 800–342–3308
Fax: 615–532–8856
Internet: www.state.tn.us/sos/statelib/lbph.htm
Hours: 8:00–4:30, M–F

State Department of Special Education

Special Education
Department of Education
Andrew Johnson Tower Eighth Floor
Nashville, TN 37247
Phone: 615–741–2851

Vocational Rehabilitation Services

Services for the Blind and Visually Impaired
Tennessee Division of Rehabilitation Services
Citizens Plaza Building 11th Floor
400 Deaderick Street
Nashville, TN 37248
Phone: 615–313–4914

National Federation of the Blind State Office

217 Oran Road
Knoxville, TN 37922–1820
Phone: 423–966–6940

TEXAS

NLS Regional Library

Texas State Library
Talking Book Program
PO Box 12927
Austin, TX 78711–2927
Phone: 512–463–5458
In-WATS: 800–252–9605
Fax: 512–463–5436
Internet: www.tsl.state.tx.us/TBP/TBPhome.html
Hours: 8:00–5:00, M–F

State Department of Special Education

Programs for Students with Visual Impairments
Texas Education Agency
1701 North Congress Avenue
Austin, TX 78701
Phone: 512–463–9414
Internet: www.tea.state.tx.us/special.ed/spec~main.ahtm

Vocational Rehabilitation Services

Texas Commission for the Blind
Administration Building
4800 North Lamar Boulevard

PO Box 12866
Austin, TX 78711
Phone: 512–459–2500

National Federation of the Blind State Office

6909 Rufus Drive
Austin, TX 78752–3123
Phone: 512–451–1717

Additional Resources

Dallas Lighthouse for the Blind, Inc.
4245 Office Parkway
Dallas, TX 75204
Phone: 214–821–2375

Lighthouse of Houston
3530 West Dallas Avenue
PO Box 130435
Houston, TX 77219
Phone: 713–527–9561

Taping for the Blind, Inc.
3935 Essex Lane
Houston, TX 77027
Phone: 713–622–2767

UTAH

NLS Regional Library

Utah State Library Division
Program for the Blind & Physically Handicapped
2150 South 300 West Suite 16
Salt Lake City, UT 84115–2579

Phone: 801–468–6789
In-WATS: 800–662–5540, Utah; 800–453–4293, western states
Fax: 801–468–6767
Hours: 8:00–5:00, M–F

State Department of Special Education

At Risk & Special Education
Office of Education
250 East 500 South
Salt Lake City, UT 84111
Phone: 801–538–7706

Vocational Rehabilitation Services

Utah Division of Services for the Blind and Visually Impaired
309 East 100 South
Salt Lake City, UT 84111
Phone: 801–323–4343

National Federation of the Blind State Office

8743 South 620 East
Sandy, Utah 84070–1744
Phone: 801–562–5540

VERMONT

NLS Regional Library

Vermont Department of Libraries
Special Services Unit
RR #4 Box 1870
Montpelier, VT 05602

Phone: 802–828–3273
In-WATS: 800–479–1711
Fax: 802–828–2199
Hours: 7:45–4:30, M–F

State Department of Special Education

Special Education Unit
Department of Education
120 State Street
Montpelier, VT 05620
Phone: 802–828–3067

Vocational Rehabilitation Services

Division for the Blind & Visually Impaired
Vermont Agency of Human Services
103 South Main Street Second Floor
Waterbury, VT 05671
Phone: 802–241–2210

National Federation of the Blind State Office

Sue Toolan
145 Berlin Street
Montpelier, VT 05602–3565
Phone: 802–229–0093

Additional Resources

Vermont Association for the Blind and Visually Impaired
37 Elmwood Avenue
Burlington, VT 05401
Phone: 802–863–1358

VIRGINIA

NLS Regional and Subregional Libraries

Library and Resource Center
Virginia Department for the Visually Handicapped
395 Azalea Avenue
Richmond, VA 23227–3623
Phone: 804–371–3661
In-WATS: 800–552–7015
Fax: 804–371–3508
Hours: 8:15–5:00, M–F

Access Services
Fairfax County Public Library
2501 Sherwood Hall Lane
Alexandria, VA 22306
Phone: 703–660–6943

Alexandria Library
Talking Book Service
826 Slaters Lane
Alexandria, VA 22314
Phone: 703–838–4298

Fredericksburg Area Subregional Library
Central Rappahannock Regional Library
1201 Caroline Street
Fredericksburg, VA 22401
Phone: 800–628–4807

Hampton Subregional Library for the Blind & Physically Handicapped
4207 Victoria Boulevard
Hampton, VA 23669
Phone: 757–727–1900

Library for the Blind & Physically Handicapped
Newport News Public Library System
110 Main Street
Newport News, VA 23601
Phone: 757–591–4858

Roanoke City Public Library
Outreach Services MeIrose-Outreach Branch
2607 Salem Turnpike NW
Roanoke, VA 24017–5397
Phone: 540–853–2648

Special Services Library
Virginia Beach Public Library
930 Independence Boulevard
Virginia Beach, VA 23455
Phone: 757–464–9175

Talking Book Center
Staunton Public Library
1 Churchville Avenue
Staunton, VA 24401
Phone: 800–995–6215

Talking Book Service
Arlington County Department of Libraries
1015 North Quincy Street
Arlington, VA 22201
Phone: 703–358–6333

State Department of Special Education

Virginia Department for the Visually Handicapped
Program for Infants, Children, and Youth
395 Azalea Avenue
Richmond, VA 23227
Phone: 804–371–3140

Vocational Rehabilitation Services

Virginia Department for the Visually Handicapped
Program for Infants, Children, and Youth
395 Azalea Avenue
Richmond, VA 23227
Phone: 804–371–3140

National Federation of the Blind State Office

6563 Williamsburg Boulevard
Arlington, VA 22213–1335
Phone: 703–534–0747

VIRGIN ISLANDS

NLS Regional Library

Virgin Islands Library for the Visually & Physically Handi-
  capped
3012 Golden Rock
Christiansted, St. Croix, VI 00820
Phone: 809–772–2250
Fax: 809–772–3545
Hours: 8:00–5:00, M–F

Department of Special Education

State Office of Special Education
Department of Education
44–46 Kongens Gade
St. Thomas, VI 00802
Phone: 809–774–4399

Vocational Rehabilitation Services

Disability & Rehabilitation Services
Department of Human Services
Knud Hansen Complex Building A
1303 Hospital Grounds
St. Thomas, VI 00802
Phone: 809–774–0930

WASHINGTON

NLS Regional Library

Washington Talking Book and Braille Library
821 Lenora Street
Seattle, WA 98121–2783
Phone: 206–464–6930
In-WATS: 800–542–0866
Fax: 206–464–0247
Internet: www.spl.lib.wa.us/wtbbl/wtbbl.html
Hours: 8:30–5:00, M–F; 9:00–1:00, Sat

State Department of Special Education

Director of Special Education
PO Box 47200
Olympia, WA 98504–7200
Phone: 360–753–6733

Vocational Rehabilitation Services

Washington State Department of Services for the Blind
1400 South Evergreen Park Drive Suite 100
Olympia, WA 98504–0933
Phone: 360–586–1224

National Federation of the Blind State Office

301 Northeast 107th Street
Vancouver, WA 98685–5340
Phone: 360–574–8221

Additional Resources

The Lighthouse for the Blind, Inc.
2501 Plum Street
PO Box C-14119
Seattle, WA 98114
Phone: 206–322–4200

WEST VIRGINIA

NLS Regional and Subregional Libraries

West Virginia Library Commission
Services for the Blind & Physically Handicapped
Cultural Center
1900 Kanawha Boulevard East
Charleston, WV 25305
Phone: 304–558–4061
In-WATS: 800–642–8674
Fax: 304–558–4066
Internet: www.wvlc.wvnet.edu/blind/bphhp.html
Hours: 8:45–5:00, M–F

Ohio County Public Library
Services for the Blind & Physically Handicapped
52 16th Street
Wheeling, WV 26003–3696
Phone: 304–232–0244

Services for the Blind & Physically Handicapped
Cabell County Public Library

455 Ninth Street Plaza
Huntington, WV 25701
Phone: 304–528–5700

Services for Blind & Physically Handicapped
Kanawha County Public Library
123 Capitol Street
Charleston, WV 25301
Phone: 304–343–4646, ext. 264

Services for the Blind & Physically Handicapped
Parkersburg and Wood County Public Library
3100 Emerson Avenue
Parkersburg, WV 26104–2414
Phone: 800–642–8674

West Virginia School for the Blind Library
301 East Main Street
Romney, WV 26757
Phone: 304–822–4894

State Department of Special Education

Special Education
Department of Education
1900 Kanawha Boulevard East Building 6
Charleston, WV 25305
Phone: 304–558–2696

Vocational Rehabilitation Services

Division of Rehabilitation Services
West Virginia State Board of Rehabilitation
State Capitol Complex
PO Box 50890
Charleston, WV 25305
Phone: 304–766–4799

National Federation of the Blind State Office

1200 Lynmar Street Number 8
Keyser, WV 26726
Phone: 304–788–0129

WISCONSIN

NLS Regional Library

Wisconsin Regional Library for the Blind & Physically Handicapped
813 West Wells Street
Milwaukee, WI 53233–1436
Phone: 414–286–3045
In-WATS: 800–242–8822
Fax: 414–286–3102
Internet: badger.state.wi.us/agencies/dpi/dlcl/goal4.htm
Hours: 8:15–4:45, M–F

State Department of Special Education

Division for Learning, Support, Equity, & Advocacy
Department of Public Instruction
125 South Webster Street
PO Box 7841
Madison, WI 53707
Phone: 608–266–1781

Vocational Rehabilitation Services

Bureau for Sensory Disabilities
Wisconsin Division of Supportive Living
2917 International Lane

PO Box 7852
Madison, WI 53707–7852
Phone: 608–243–5622

National Federation of the Blind State Office

5331 South Eighth Street
Milwaukee, WI 53221–3625
Phone: 414–483–3336

WYOMING

NLS Regional Library

Wyoming readers receive library service from the NLS library
in Salt Lake City, Utah.

State Department of Special Education

Special Education
Department of Education
Hathaway Building
2300 Capitol Avenue
Cheyenne, WY 82002
Phone: 307–777–6257

Vocational Rehabilitation Services

Vocational Rehabilitation Division
Department of Employment
Herschler Building
Cheyenne, WY 82002
Phone: 307–777–7385

National Federation of the Blind State Office

428 West 12th Street
Casper, WY 82601–4106
Phone: 307–237–7798

U.S. CITIZENS ABROAD

U.S. citizens residing in foreign countries receive library service from:

Network Services Section
National Library for the Blind & Physically Handicapped
Library of Congress
Washington, DC 20542
Phone: 202–707–9261
Fax: 202–707–0712
Internet: www.loc.gov/nls
Hours: 8:00–4:30, M–F

Appendix B: Commercial Audio Publishers

Why buy recorded books that you can usually borrow for free from Recording for the Blind & Dyslexic or the National Library Service? Simple: it is sometimes the fastest way to get a book, which makes it a viable reading solution. Even a rush delivery from RFB&D takes days, while a credit card and overnight shipping can have a book at your door in a matter of hours. New titles are available more quickly from commercial vendors than from RFB&D or the NLS. They can be played on all cassette players, and usually feature the highest production values of any recordings. And, of course, they're yours to keep, so you can build a library, or recycle to friends or the local library, where you will no doubt find an ever-expanding audio section. The main criteria for this list were companies publishing unabridged works, and titles germane to school and college curriculums. There are, however, nearly 3,000 commercial publishers and professional organizations producing tapes on virtually every subject, occupation, hobby, and endeavor. This list should get you started. If a company interests you, give them a call, ask for a catalog, and get on their mailing list. Visit their website, download any clips that interest you, and let them know what you want. Many publishers offer discounts for the sight-impaired, as well as good introductory offers.

Academic Success Press
PO Box 25002
Bradenton, FL 34206
Phone: 941–359–2819
Fax: 941–753–2882
Internet: www.bookmasters.com
  Products developed by Dr. Paul Notling focusing on improving math and test-taking skills. Titles include: *Winning at Math Success Kit, How to Reduce Test Anxiety, How to Ace Tests.*

Adventures in Cassettes
5353 Nathan Lane North
Plymouth, MN 55442–1978
Toll free: 800–328–0108
Fax: 612–553–0424
Internet: www.aic-radio.com
  Great selection of old-time radio, including mysteries, comedy, and drama, many nice boxed sets. Includes *The Shadow, Boston Blackie, The Green Hornet, The Whistler, The Saint*, and many more.

Airplay Audio Publishing
972 Lexington Avenue
New York, NY 10021
Phone: 800–459–4925
Fax: 212–879–1013
Internet: www.airplayaudio.com
  Specializes in high-quality, unabridged popular works read by world-famous actors. Titles include: *Trojan Gold* by Elizabeth Peters, read by Kathleen Turner; *The Story of Doctor Dolittle* by Hugh Lofting, read by Martin Short; *The Complete Shakespeare Sonnets* by William Shakespeare, read by various actors, including Tony Randall and Eli Wallach.

American Audio Prose Library
PO Box 842

Columbia, MO 65205
Phone: 573–443–0361
Toll free: 800–447–2275
Fax: 573–499–0579

Specializes in recordings by American writers reading and discussing their works. Titles include: Annie Dillard reads "Total Eclipse" (essay) from her collection *Teaching a Stone to Talk*, John Yount reads two chapters from *Hardcastle*.

Audio Book Contractors
Classic Books on Cassettes
PO Box 40115
Washington, DC 20016–0115
Phone: 202–363–3429
Fax: 202–363–3429

Comprehensive collection of complete classics on tape. Titles include: *A Collection of Haunting Tales, Some Tame Gazelle* by Barbara Pym, *Three Tales* by Flaubert.

Audio Books on Compact Disc, Inc.
5161 Staverly Lane
Norcross, Georgia 30092
Phone: 770–446–1100
Toll free: 888–749–6342
Fax: 770–417–1242

The most complete inventory of audiobooks recorded in CD format, including fiction, nonfiction, poetry, and drama.

The Audio Bookshelf Collection
174 Prescott Hill Road
Northport, Maine 04849
Toll free: 800–234–1713
Internet: www.agate.net/~audbkshf/index.html

This company sells multi-title samplers or theme packages, such as "Broadening the Mind," featuring 17 titles, including Einstein's *Relativity*, Henry James' *The Art of the Novel*, and works by Descartes and Simone de Beauvoir. You can buy tapes separately as well. Titles include: *Writing Seinfield Style, The Hobbit, The Art of Mingling.*

Audio Editions
Books on Cassette
PO Box 6930
Auburn, CA 95603
Phone: 916–888–7803
Toll free: 800–231–4261
Fax: 800–882–1840
Internet: www.audioeditions.com

Audio Editions has a wide variety of recorded books, both abridged and unabridged, including fiction, nonfiction, self-help, business, and humor. Titles include: *To Kill a Mockingbird* by Harper Lee; *The Best of Car Talk, Mastering a Foreign Language.*

Audio Forum
The Language Source
96 Broad Street
Guilford, CT 06437
Phone: 203–453–9794
Toll free: 800–243–1234
Fax: 203–453–9774
Internet: http://agoralang.com/audioforum.html

Specializes in foreign language cassettes, CD-ROMs, and other learning materials. Also has a Cassette-of-the-Month Club. Titles include: Basic French Conversation, French Radio Commercials Word-a-Day calendars. Features many languages, including Arabic, Apache, and Urdu.

Audio Literature Presents
370 West San Bruno Avenue
San Bruno, CA 94066
Toll free: 800–383–0174
Fax: 510–559–1629

Great selection of contemporary literature, including nonfiction, poetry, Native Americans, spiritual classics, inspiration, and biography. Titles include: *Great Books* by David Denby, *Letters to a Young Poet* by Rainer Maria Rilke, *The Basketball Diaries* by Jim Carroll.

Audio Partners Publishing
PO Box 6930
Auburn, CA 95603–6930
Toll free: 800–231–4261
Fax: 800–882–1840
Internet: www.audiopartners.com

Resells many popular titles, such as the unabridged British novels from Cover to Cover (see below). They also publishes its own works and offers a wide range of popular and classic literature, as well as children's titles. Titles include: *A Night to Remember: The Titanic's Last Hour* by Walter Lord, *The Killer Angels* by Michael Shaara, *Babette's Feast & Sorrow Acre* by Isak Dinesen.

The Audio Press
PO Box 666
Niwot, CO 80544
Phone: 303–652–3050

A great resource, with tapes on Indian folklore, natural history, Save the Loons, etcetera. Titles include: *A Sense of Place* by Wallace Stegner, *Natural Acts: A Sidelong View of Science and Nature* by David Quammen, *Loon Magic* by Tom Klein.

Audio Renaissance Tapes
5858 Wilshire Boulevard Suite 200
Los Angeles, CA 90036
Phone: 213–939–1840
Toll free: 800–488–5233
Fax: 714–457–1812
Internet: www.audiosource.com/audio

Variety of popular and self-help titles by such notables as Larry King and star motivator Anthony Robbins. Titles include: *You Gotta Play Hurt* by Dan Jenkins, *On the Trail of the Assassins* by John Garrison, *Earl Nightingale's Greatest Discovery* by Earl Nightingale.

Audio Scholar
PO Box 1456
Mendocino, CA 95460
Phone: 707–937–1225
Toll free: 800–282–1225
Fax: 707–937–1869

Scholarly works from Harvard, Princeton, and MIT university presses that are, abridged. Titles include: *T. Rex and the Crater of Doom* by Walter Alvarez; *Relativity* by Albert Einstein; *Essays on Art, Nature, & Spirituality* by Ralph Waldo Emerson.

AudioText, Inc.
PO Box 418
Barker, TX 77413
Toll free: 800–860–3910
Fax: 281–398–9481
Internet: www.flash.net/~atx

Small but impressive list of science fiction short-story titles. Titles include: *Under Siege* by George R. R. Martin, *Blood Sisters* by Greg Egan, *The Shobies' Story* by Ursula K. Le Guin.

August House
PO Box 3223
Little Rock, AK 72203–3223
Phone: 501–372–5450
Toll free: 800–284–8784
Fax: 501–372–5579

Collection of tapes and books for readers of all ages, including multicultural works, world folklore, and U.S. history. Titles include: *The Grand Canyon* by Donald Davis, *Wonder Tales from Around the World* by Heather Forest, *Cajun Folk Tales* by J. J. Reneaux.

Baker & Taylor Books
2709 Water Ridge Parkway
Charlotte, NC 28217
Phone: 704–357–3500
Fax: 704–329–8989

This comprehensive distributor is one of the names to know, offering titles from numerous audio publishers, large and small. A great way for audio listeners to keep abreast of what's coming.

BDD Audio Publishing
Bantam Doubleday Dell
1540 Broadway
New York, NY 10036
Phone: 212–782–9852
Toll free: 800–223–5780
Fax: 800–233–3294

Includes full range of books produced by Bantam Audio, including Bantam Classics. Fiction includes John Grisham and Robert Ludlum. Nonfiction includes the popular "Don't Know Much About" series, with tapes on the Civil War and geography.

B&B Audio, Inc.
3175 Commercial Boulevard 107-B
Northbrook, IL 60062
Phone: 847–562–9516
Toll free: 800–3–LISTEN
Fax: 847–562–9517
Internet: www.bandbaudio.com

A mix of classics and contemporary fiction and nonfiction for readers of all ages, running the gamut from *Anne of Green Gables* to *The Godfather*. Titles include *The Secret Sharer* by Joseph Conrad, *Frank Sinatra: An American Legend* by Nancy Sinatra, *The Downing of TWA Flight 800* by James Sanders, *The Stock Market Crash of 1929* by Ann Abrams.

B.F.I. Audiobooks
1397 Hope Street
Stamford, CT 06907
Phone: 203–968–2255
Toll free: 800–260–7717

Eclectic collection of titles that range from dealing with irate people and the basics of soliciting corporate gifts, to midlife crisis stories. Also a tape on how to market your own audiobooks. Titles include: *Internet Explained—Short and Sweet, 60 Minutes towards Computer Literacy, Stalking the Corporate Dollar.*

Big Sur Tapes
P.O. Box 4-WB
Tiburon, California 94920
Phone: 415–289–5280
Toll free: 800–688–5512
Fax: 415–289–5285
Internet: www.bigsurtapes.com

Big Sur offers wisdom and sacred inspiration with its treasury of live recordings. There are many fine tapes here, including works by mythologist Joseph Campbell, poet Allen Ginsberg, Buckminster Fuller, Anna Freud, Thomas Merton, Rollo May, Henry Miller, and Abraham Maslow.

Blackstone Audio Books
PO Box 969
Ashland, OR 97520
Phone: 541–482–9294
Toll free: 800–729–2665

The single best source for unabridged classics. Titles include:

Candide by Voltaire, *Notes from the Underground* by Tolstoy, *A History of the Middle East, Napoleon and Hitler.*

BMP Audio
Suite 201-W
1440 Whalley Avenue
New Haven, CT 06515
Toll free: 800–205–8254
Fax: 800–575–0737

Small but well-wrought selection of tapes with Hellenistic appeal. Television's Hercules (Kevin Sorbo) reads tales of the young hero, and Julie Harris and Michael York read from the works of Sappho. Titles include: *Enchanted Tales*, narrators include Katharine Hepburn and Jason Robards; *Sappho—Touched by Eros* by Julie Harris and Michael York; *Hercules, and Young Hercules* by Kevin Sorbo.

Bookcassette Sales
PO Box 481
Grand Haven, MI 49417
Toll free: 800–222–3225
Fax: 616–846–0630

All uncut, mainstream titles, from Molly Ivins comedic commentaries to James Bond novels. Frequent discounts. Titles include: *Blood Work* by Michael Connelly, *Cavedweller* by Dorothy Allison, *Uncle Tom's Cabin* by Harriot Beecher Stowe.

Books in Motion
9212 East Montgomery
Suite 501
Spokane, WA 99206
Phone: 509–922–1646
Toll free: 800–752–3199
Fax: 509–922–1445

Great selection of popular books, including westerns, mystery, fantasy, all unabridged. Has children's books, too, as well as The Commuter Collection. Titles include: *Treasure Island* by Robert Louis Stevenson, *A White Heron and Three Other Stories* by Sarah Orne Jewett, *The Call of the Wild* by Jack London.

Books on Tape
PO Box 7900
Newport Beach, CA 92658
Phone: 714–548–5525
Toll free: 800–626–3333

It has a 256-page catalog, which contains 5,000 books for rent only. Wide selection.

Brilliance Audio
PO Box 887
1704 Eaton Drive
Grand Haven, MI 49417
Phone: 616–846–5256
Toll free: 800–648–2312
Fax: 616–846–0630
Internet: www.brillianceaudio.com

Audiobook publisher/distributor specializing in unabridged bestsellers on cassette. Over 500 bestselling fiction and nonfiction audiobook titles, simultaneous release with hardcover.

Caedmon
HarperAudio
10 East 53rd Street
New York, NY 10022
Phone: 212–207–6905
Toll free: 800–242–7737

Perhaps the best source for classic literature on cassette, including plays, poetry, and fiction. Your school or public library is likely stocked with Caedmon titles. Titles range from Plato, to Shakespeare, to Philip Roth with the occasional popular title, such as rock star Jewel's first book of poems.

Chivers Audio Books
Box 1450
Hampton, NH 03843–1450
Toll free: 800–704–2005
Fax: 603–929–3890

Solid selection of unabridged audio titles for rent or purchase, including both popular and classic works, mystery, science fiction, and romance. Titles include: *Odds Against* by Dick Francis, *The Martian Chronicles* by Ray Bradbury, *Buffalo Girls* by Larry McMurtry.

CIL Publications
Visions
500 Greenwich Street
New York, NY 10013
Toll free: 888–255–8333
Internet: www.cilpubs.com

Small but important list of books on mobility, sensory development, and personal management for those who are losing their sight or who are already blind, developed by a team of top rehabilitation experts. Titles include: *Indoor Mobility Audiobook, Personal Management Audiobook, Housekeeping Audiobook.*

Cover to Cover Cassettes
PO Box 112
Marlborough
Wilshire SN8 3UG
Phone: 44–(0)–264–731227
Fax: 44–(0)–264–731390

Unabridged Jane Austin or George Elliot novels. Great narrators. Titles include: *Middlemarch* by George Eliot, *Emma* by Jane Austin, *Oliver Twist* by Charles Dickens.

Dercum Audio
3356 Coffey Lane

Santa Rosa, CA 95403
Distributed by Associated Publishers Group
1501 County Hospital Road
Nashville, TN 37218
Phone: 707–541–3333
Toll free: 800–327–5113
Fax: 707–542–4444
Internet: www.bookbase.com/dercum

Great series of horror, science fiction, and other genre fiction, such as adventure, romance, and children's books.

Dove Audio
855 Beverly Boulevard
Los Angeles, CA 90048
Phone: 310–786–1600
Toll free: 800–368–3007
Fax: 310–247–2924
Internet: www.doveaudio.com

Many of this publisher's popular titles are abridged but have high production values. The catalog is ever-expanding. Includes popular novelists such as Sidney Sheldon and Jacqueline Suzanne, and a selection of popular poetry, business, and self-help titles. Titles include: *A Brief History of Time* by Stephen Hawking, *Terms of Success: More Word Workout for a Stronger Vocabulary* by Jeffrey McQuain, *Fifty Poems of Emily Dickinson* read by such luminaries as Glenda Jackson and Sharon Stone.

Durkin Hayes Publishing
One Columbia Drive
Niagra Falls, NY 14305
Phone: 716–298–5150
Toll free: 800–962–5200
Fax: 716–298–5607

Most of the books here are abridged, but the catalog is nicely made and full of popular titles including Isaac Asimov, Stephen

King, and Ellery Queen. Titles include: *The Monkey's Paw and Other Tales of Terror, The Invisible Man* by H. G. Wells, *Dracula* by Bram Stoker.

Earbooks
PO Box 976
Camden, ME 04843–0976
Phone: 207–236–3771
Internet: www.midcoast.com/~earbooks/
   Small, eclectic collection of original audio books with a Maine flavor, some of which carry original musical accompaniment. Includes motivational material. Titles include: *The Moose Who Wanted to Be a Reindeer & Luke and the Christmas Dragon* by Ned Ackerman, *Financial Pot of Goals* by Dorothy O'Donnell.

G. K. Hall
1633 Broadway, 5th Floor
New York, NY 10019
Phone: 212–702–6789
Toll free: 800–257–5755
   Selection of popular children's and adult titles, with a scattering of classics, all fiction. Titles include: *Charlie and the Great Glass Elevator* by Roald Dahl, *Mortimer Says Nothing* by Joan Aiken, *Joy in the Morning* by P. G. Wodehouse.

Global Fearon
4350 Equity Drive
Columbus, OH 43216
Toll free: 800–877–4283
   Unique educational sets on science and math, and programs to teach life skills and vocations.

HarperAudio
HarperCollins Publishers
10 East 53rd Street
New York, NY 10022

Phone: 212–207–7000
Toll free: 800–242–7757
Fax: 800–822–4090
Internet: www.harpercollins.com

Major audio publisher. Includes Caedmon imprint, which has the best selection of the highest-quality literature of any publisher. Caedmon also has tapes on African-American interests, business, humor, philosophy, sports, and the classics. HarperAudio features titles on business as well as novelizations of *The X Files Movie.*

Hear and Know
1741 Decree Avenue
West Columbia, SC 29169
Phone: 803–796–4887
Fax: 803–796–4887

Specializes in cassette tutorials on a variety of computer topics, including Windows, Corel, WordPerfect, Real Audio, DOS, and many others.

High Windy Audio
PO Box 553
Fairview, NC 28730
Phone: 704–628–1728
Toll free: 800–637–8679

Selection of tapes for parents of young children, including one title on how to get your child to sleep, by a *Family Circle* columnist, and some story collections.

JinCim Recordings
PO Box 536
Portsmouth, RI 02871
Phone: 401–847–5148
Toll free: 800–538–3034
Internet: www.jincim.com

One of the oldest commercial audio publishers, offering stories for readers young and old, including many classics of American and English literature as well as essays, biography, genre fiction, and world literature. Website features free stories. Titles include: *Emma* by Jane Austen, *Zen and the Art of the Internet* by Brendan Keyhoe, "The Adventure of the Gloria Scott" by Arthur Conan Doyle.

Knowledge Products
PO Box 305151
Nashville, TN 37230
Phone: 615–742–3852
Toll free: 800–876–4332

Famous for its Audio Classics series, which includes *The Giants of Philosophers* (24 cassettes), *The Great Economic Thinkers, Secrets of the Great Inventors, Science & Discovery*, and *The Giants of Political Thought*. All are narrated by notables such as Charlton Heston, Edwin Newman, and Lynn Redgrave.

LA Theatre Works
Attn: Tape Department
681 Venice Boulevard
Venice, CA 90291
Phone: 310–827–0889
Fax: 310–827–4949
Internet: www.kcrw.org/latw/latw.html

Audio versions of the theater's productions range from *Julius Caesar* to Neil Simon's *Brighton Beach Memoirs*. Also included are dramatizations of novels, such as the Graham Greene's classic, *The Third Man*, and famous Scopes monkey trial, based on court transcripts. The actors include some of the best, such as Jason Alexander, Julie Harris, and Charles Derning.

Learn, Incorporated
113 Gaither Drive
Mt. Laurel, NJ 08054–9987
Phone: 800–729–7323

Fine set of goal-achieving and speed-learning cassette programs called Smart Tapes. Titles include: *Goof-Proof Grammar, Being in the Zone, Winning Vocabulary, Go for Your
Goals.*

Library of Congress
Motion Picture, Broadcasting,
and Recorded Sound Division
Public Services Office
101 Independence Avenue, SE
Washington, DC 20540
Phone: 202–707–5093
Internet: www.library of congress.gov

In addition to its array of NLS services, the Library of Congress sells many types of audio recordings from its Motion Picture, Broadcasting, and Recorded Sound Division, including
folk and chamber music, poetry and literature in both English
and Spanish. Titles include: *Nine Pulitzer Prize Poets Read
Their Own Poems,* Trio in Eb for Clarinet, Viola, and Piano—
Mozart performed by American Chamber Players.

Listen & Live Audio
PO Box 817
Roseland, NJ 07068
Toll free: 800–653–9400
Fax: 201–798–3225
Internet: www.listenandlive.com

What this publisher lacks in titles it more than makes up for
in obscurity, with such topics as a wrap-up of the 1993–1994
Wisconsin football season. Titles include: *Don't Sweat the
Small Stuff* by Michael R. Mantell, *Maintaining Balance during
Loss and Beyond* by Diane Chapman, *What Do Women Want
from Men?* by Dan True.

Listening Library
One Park Avenue

Old Greenwich, CT 06970–1727
Phone: 203–637–1839
Toll free: 800–243–4504
Fax: 800–454–0606

Wide variety of children's and adult titles, including *The Outsiders* by S. E. Hinton and *Are You There God, It's Me, Margaret*. Adult titles include: Hemmingway and Fitzgerald story collections, *Heart of Darkness* by Joseph Conrad, and *The Metamorphous* by Franz Kafka.

Listen-to-Learn Audiotapes
4500 East 9th Avenue
Denver, CO 80220
Phone: 303–452–7643
Toll free: 800–919–8899
Fax: 303–255–9050

Collection from psychologist Susan Heitler includes tapes on conflict resolution, anxiety, and depression. Titles include: *The Power of Two, Anxiety—Friend or Foe? Depression—A Disorder of Power*.

Live Oak Media
PO Box 652
Pine Plains, NY 12567
Phone: 518–398–1010
Fax: 518–398–1070

Focuses on "readalong" books and filmstrips for young readers, and has many classics such as Ludwig Bemelmans' *Madeline* series, and Nancy Carlson's series on *Harriet the Hippo*, with sets that include book and cassette.

Lodes Tone
611 Empire Mill Road
Bloomington, IN 47401
Phone: 812–824–2400
Toll free: 800–411–6563

Fax: 812–824–2401

Internet: www.lodestone-media.com

This company specializes in "movies for your mind," riding the retro wave of interest in audio theater. Titles include H. G. Wells' *War of the Worlds*, and Bram Stoker's *Dracula*, as well as more recent productions in a variety of genres, including comedy, mystery, and science fiction.

Luna Media

4107 Laguna Street

Coral Gables, Florida 33146

Fax: 305–447–4643

The Mind's Eye

Memory Lane

Chelmsford, MA 01824–0947

Toll free: 800–949–3333

Fax: 800–866–3235

Its nostalgia gift catalog, features tapes, including comedy, old-time radio mysteries, and classics.

National Audio Theater

PO Box 933

Hendersonville, NC 28739

Internet: www.wncguide.com/nat

The Blue Ridge Radio Players produce audio plays and distribute them free to the sight-impaired through most NLS regional libraries. Their website tells which libraries have them. They also sell tapes to the general public for a small fee. Titles include: *An Occurrence at Owl Creek Bridge* by Ambrose Bierce, *The Red-Headed League* by Arthur Conan Doyle, *Gift of the Magi* by O. Henry.

National Recording Company

PO Box 395

Glenview, IL 60025
Phone: 407–282–3489
   Wealth of old-time radio broadcasts.

New Leaf Distributing Company
401 Thornton Road
Lithia Springs, GA 30122–1557
Phone: 800–326–2665
Fax: 800–326–1066
Internet: www.newleaf-dist.com
   Along with Baker & Taylor, this is a major distributor of spoken audio, specializing in the harmonious development of human potential. Topics include African heritage and wisdom, Native American studies, Chinese philosophy and Taoism, folklore and fairy tales, journal writing, mind power, wellness, creativity, and humor. Also has wide selection of biographies, fiction, poetry, and young adult books.

New World Library
14 Pamaron Way
Novato, CA 94949
Toll free: 800–972–6657
Fax: 415–884–2199
Internet: www.nwlib.com
   This publisher's audio titles focus on motivation and life fulfillment. Great catalog. Titles include: *You Can Be Happy No Matter What* (abridged) by Dr. Richard Carlson, *The Seven Spiritual Laws of Success* by Deepak Chopra, *Creating True Prosperity* by Shakti Gawain.

Nightingale-Conant
7300 North Lehigh Avenue
Niles, IL 60714
Phone: 647–647–0300
Toll free: 800–525–9000
   A complete selection of motivational tape sets, including the

work of founder Earl Nightingale (*The Strangest Secret*), Zig Ziglar (*See You At the Top*), Denis Waitley (*The Course in Winning*), and many more.

Oral Tradition Archives
PO Box 51155
Pacific Grove, CA 93950
Phone: 408–663–1682
Toll free: 800–779–1116
Fax: 408–663–0500
   Tape sets by storytellers Michael Meade and Marian Woodman, and seminars including psychologist James Hillman. Personal growth, mythology, men's movement. Titles include: *Men and the Life of Desire* with Meade, Hillman, and Robert Bly; *Chaos or Creativity* by Marion Woodman; *The Dance of Gender* by Michael Meade.

Pacifica Radio Archives
PO Box 8092 Dept. B
Universal City, CA 91608–0092
Phone: 818–506–1077
Toll free: 800–735–0230
Fax: 818–506–1084
   Radio interviews with political thinkers and writers, including Henry Miller, Alice Walker, James Baldwin, and Muhammad Ali. Great resource for research.

Pegasus Concepts
PO Box 1933
Mountain Home, AR 72654
Phone: 870–491–5040
Toll free: 800–968–5036
Fax: 870–491–5041
Internet: www.pegasusbooks.com
   Internet audio store featuring the full sweep of human experience, from the classics to 91 titles on *Star Wars* and *Star*

Trek. Their site also maintains a sale bin. Titles include: *Stepping Stones* by Seamus Heaney, *Death of a Salesman* by Arthur Miller, *The Outsiders* by S. E. Hinton.

Pelican Publishing Company
1101 Monroe Street
PO Box 3110
Gretna, LA 70054
Phone: 504–368–1175
Toll free: 800–843–1724
Fax: 504–368–1195
Internet: www.pelicanpub.com

A fine general publisher specializing in Southern history offers children's holiday and educational titles with local color. Titles include: *Cajun Night before Christmas* by Colleen Salley and the Clovis Crawfish series, that feature lessons and stories in French and English.

A. W. Peller & Associates
Educational Materials
210 Sixth Avenue
PO Box 106
Hawthorne, NJ 07507–0106
Phone: 973–423–4666
Toll free: 800–451–7450
Fax: 973–423–5569
Internet: www.awpeller.com

Produces works in various media mainly for teachers and librarians, but be sure to peruse the catalog, which includes read-along book and cassette packages, videos, and curriculum-related CD-ROMs. Titles include: *Walk Two Moons* by Sharon Creech, *The Pinballs* by Betsy Byars. Also distributes *January Productions Mystery Readalongs* and *People to Remember* series.

Penguin Audio
Penguin USA
375 Hudson Street

New York, NY 10014
Phone: 201–387–0600
Toll free: 800–526–0275
Fax: 800–227–9604

Major publisher of audio texts on a wide variety of subjects, both popular and classic. Titles include: *101 Great Answers to the Toughest Interview Questions* by Ron Fry; *On the Road* by Jack Kerouac; *Animal Farm* by George Orwell; *At Dawn We Slept*, and *The Bambino* by Dan Shaughnessy.

Penton Overseas
2470 Impala Drive
Carlsbad, CA 92008
Phone: 760–431–0060
Toll free: 800–748–5804
Fax: 760–431–8110
Internet: www.pentonoverseas.com

Source of foreign language study guides on cassette and CD-ROM. Also sells a wide range of audiobooks through its website.

Plays on Tape
P.O. Box 5789
Bend, OR 97708–5789
Phone: 541–923–6246
Toll free: 800–752–9974
Fax: 541–923–9679
Internet: www.playsontape.com

This company produces audio theater on tape and CD-ROM.

Poet's Audio Center
6925 Willow Street NW Suite 201
Washington, DC 20012–2023
Phone: 202–722–9105
Toll free: 800–366–9105
Fax: 202–722–9106
Internet: www.writer.org/pac/pac01.htm

Their specialty is poets reading their own works, and nearly every noteworthy modern poet is represented, from T. S. Eliot, to the more recent poets. Titles include: *In Their Own Voices: A Century of Recorded Poetry, The Diaries of Anais Nin, Poetry and Reflections* by Langston Hughes.

Prelude Press
8165 Mannix Drive
Los Angeles, CA 90046
Phone: 213–650–9571
Toll free: 800–543–3101

Motivational packages—ones you might rent at your local library. Titles include: *Life 101* by John-Roger and Peter McWilliams, *You Can't Afford the Luxury of a Negative Thought* and *Do It! Let's Get off Our Butts*.

Publisher's Group West
4065 Hollis Street
Emeryville, CA 94608
Phone: 510–658–3453
Toll free: 800–788–3123

Nice catalog with solid selection of contemporary fiction and nonfiction read by famous actors. Titles include: *Humor on Wry* a three-tape anthology, *Under the Garden* by Graham Greene, read by Derek Jacobi.

The Publishing Mills AudioBooks
9220 Sunset Boulevard, Suite 302
Los Angeles, CA 90069
Toll free: 800–722–8346
Fax: 213–858–5391
Internet: www.pubmills.com

Fairly large selection covering a variety of popular interests, from Diane Ackerman's *Natural History of Love* to the Nixon-Kennedy debates. Titles include: *All You Need to Know about the Music Business* by Donald S. Passman, *Deadly Evolution:*

The Virulence of Viruses by The Smithsonian Institution, *Friday Night Lights* by H. G. Bissinger, *Griffin & Sabine Trilogy* by Nick Bantock.

Random House Audio
201 East 50th Street, 22nd Floor
New York, NY 10022
Phone: 212–751–2600
Toll free: 800–726–0600

Lots of abridged titles, such as *Fried Green Tomatoes at the Whistle Stop Cafe* by Fanny Flagg, *Amazing Grace* by Judy Collins.

The Reader's Chair
Box 2626
Hollister, CA 95024
Toll free: 800–616–1350
Fax: 408–636–1296
Internet: www.readerschair.com

Company produces unabridged, award-winning sci-fi stories with a little mystery and suspense thrown in. Titles include: *Falling Free* by Lois McMaster Bujold, *Hideaway* by Dean Koontz, *Murder on the Run* by Gloria White.

Recorded Books
270 Skipjack Road
Prince Frederick, MD 20678
Phone: 410–535–5590
Toll free: 800–638–1304
Fax: 410–535–5499

Over 2,000 unabridged titles for sale or 30-day rental. Website also rents on-line. Great catalog. Titles include: *West with the Night* by Beryl Markham, *The Jews: Story of a People* by Howard Fast, *Midnight in the Garden of Good and Evil* by John Berendt.

Second Renaissance Books
143 West Street
New Milford, CT 06776
Phone: 860–354–5448
Toll free: 800–729–6149
Fax: 860–355–7160
Internet: www.rationalmind.com
   Though this publisher mainly promotes the work of philosopher Ayn Rand, there are some other titles here, including: *Principals of Grammar, Introduction to Logic*, and an omnibus set *The History of Philosophy*.

Simon & Schuster
200 Old Tappan Road
Old Tappan, NJ 07675
Toll free: 800–223–2336
Fax: 800–445–6991
   A wide selection of titles, from vocabulary builders to popular genres. Includes a wealth of *Star Trek* books, both Kirk and Picard.

Smithsonian Associates
MRC 701
1100 Jefferson Drive SW
Washington, DC 20560
Phone: 202–357–3030
Fax: 202–786–2034
Internet: www.si.edu/youandsi/join/tsa/abouttsa.htm
   Great set of live recordings of presentations at the Smithsonian, which offer entertainment as well as unique primary sources for research papers. Titles include: "Adapting Shakespeare for Film" by Kenneth Branagh, "The Imaginable Future" by Bill Gates, "A Lifetime Reporting the News" by Walter Cronkite, "Criminal Justice after the O. J. Simpson Case" by Alan Dershowitz.

SOUNDELUX Audio Publishing
37 Commercial Boulevard
Novato, CA 94949
Phone: 415–883–7701
Internet: www.soundelux.com

Formerly The Mind's Eye, this company pioneered audio literature for the general public in 1971, offering classics like A Baker Street Dozen by Arthur Conan Doyle, and the J.R.R. Tolkien Rings Trilogy. Titles include: *A Book of American Humor* by Russell Baker, *Truman: A Journey to Independence* by David McCullough.

Sounds True
PO Box 8010
Boulder, CO 80306–8010
Phone: 303–665–3151
Toll free: 800–333–9185
Fax: 303–665–5292

A large selection of tapes on the human spirit, creativity, men's and women's issues, anger, and healing. Works by Robert Bly, Thich Nhat Hanh, Clarissa Pinkola Estes, and many others. Titles include: *The Energy of Money* by Maria Nemeth, *The Science of Enlightenment* by Shinzen Young, *Vocal Awareness* by Arthur Joseph.

Spectrum Audio Text
PO Box 131
Wantagh, NY 11793
Toll free: 800–382–0679, ext. 133

Tapes for those who want to travel, or who want the sights and stories. Titles include: *Taking the Mystery out of American Wine, Around and About New York City and Long Island, New York Weekends—More or Less.*

The Spoken Arts
801 94th Avenue North

St. Petersburg, FL 33702
Toll free: 800–326–4090
Fax: 813–578–3110

Great selection of children's titles, as well as world literature, poetry, drama, and history. Titles include: *The Man Who Mistook His Wife for a Hat* by Oliver Sacks, *The Secret Garden* by Frances Hodgson Burnett, *A Child's Garden of Verses* by Robert Louis Stevenson.

Tangled Web Audio
3380 Sheridan Drive, Suite 167
Amherst, NY 14226
Phone: 519–442–5010
Fax: 519–442–2346
Internet: www.nas.net/~tangled/

Specializes in mystery and suspense, and features several tape anthologies. Titles include: *Hauntings: A Classic Collection* which includes tales by Robert Louis Stevenson and Washington Irving, *A Vampyre Story* by J. Sheridan Le Fanu; *Vintage Crime Stories*, which includes stories from British greats Graham Greene and Margery Allingham.

The Teaching Company
7405 Alban Station Court Suite A107
Springfield, VA 22150–2318
Phone: 800–832–2412
Fax: 703–912–7756

This catalog sells audio and videocassette copies of complete courses by "superstar teachers." Courses range from basic math to understanding Einstein. Titles include: *How to Become a SuperStar Student, How to Understand and Listen to Great Music, Cosmic Questions: Astronomy from Quark to Quasar.*

Ten Speed Press
PO Box 7123

Berkeley, CA 94707
Toll free: 800–841–BOOK
   Great classics such as *Black Elk Speaks*, Rilke's *Letters to a Young Poet*, and *A Separate Reality*.

Time Warner Audiobooks
9229 Sunset Boulevard 8th floor
Los Angeles, CA 90069
(Distributed by Time-Warner Books, NY)
Phone: 310–204–7421
Internet: pathfinder.com/twep/twab
   Most of the titles are abridged, and some are audio versions of Time-Life book series. Titles include: (All unabridged) *Health Journeys: Diabetes* by Belleruth Naparstek, *The Chase: Strange Highways Collection* by Dean Koontz, *Voices of the Civil War: Soldier Life* by Time-Life Books with John Whitman. The company also publishes a set of classic study guides, which include a copy of the book and a cassette of excerpts and questions.

Trafalgar Square
PO Box 257
Howe Hill Road
North Pomfret, VT 05053
Phone: 800–423–4525
Fax: 802–457–1913
Internet: www.trafalgarsquarebooks.com
   Publishes numerous audiobooks for children and adults, including fiction, poetry and drama, religious works, and classics.

Ulverscroft Soundings
279 Boston Street
Guilford, CT 06437
Phone: 203–453–2080
Toll free: 800–955–9659
   Great selection of tapes and large-print books. Includes many classics.

Village Story Tapes
937 Midpine Way
PO Box 1440
Sebastopol, CA 95473–1440
Phone: 800–238–8273
Fax: 707–823–1128
Internet: www.vstapes.com

This is a service-oriented Internet reseller with over 1,000 titles for sale or rent in a wide array of genres. One of the better web storefronts that includes a search engine. Titles include: *Alias Grace* by Margaret Atwood, *Like Water for Chocolate* by Laura Esquivel, *Snow Falling on Cedars* by David Guterson.

Wireless
Minnesota Public Radio
PO Box 64454
St. Paul, MN 55115
Toll free: 800–733–3369
Fax: 612–645–7092
Internet: www.mpr.org

Classical music, self-improvement, vintage radio, Garrison Keillor, Stephen King, and a few full-length books.

Yellow Moon Press
PO Box 381316
Cambridge, MA 02238
Phone: 617–776–2230
Toll free: 800–497–4385
Fax: 617–776–8246

Yellow Moon specializes in preserving and enhancing the oral tradition, particularly in storytelling, with titles from the field's top practitioners. Titles include: *For Younger I've Been— Stories of a Belfast Childhood* by Maggie Peirce, *Ghostly Tales of Japan* by Rafe Martin, *Folktales of Strong Women* by Doug Lipman.

Appendix C: What to Read— 60 for Starters

No matter which "Great Books" list inspires you, all titles are available in many formats.

No education is faster and longer lasting than what you create for yourself by reading the world's great books. Since the phrase "great books" often sparks more controversy than reading, we present 60 titles from three established and well-respected lists that are intended as points of departure for your journey into books.

The American Library Association's "Outstanding Books for the College Bound," Robert B. Downs's *Books That Changed the World*, and the compilation of the Great Books Society (University of Chicago) have their particular slants, but each lists books that have made an impact on society and culture, marking either supreme literary accomplishment or vital crossroads in the history of human thought and culture. Most still affect to some degree how we perceive the world and how today's writers and thinkers portray humanity.

The bibliography provides a selection from each list, arranged alphabetically, and tells where to obtain each in the specialized formats of cassette, large print, and braille.

Each entry includes the Recording for the Blind & Dyslexic shelf number, the NLS cassette number, a braille identification number (most of which are produced for the NLS), and mention of the availability of large-print or commercial audio versions, on either cassette or CD-ROM. Information on all audio publishers, whose works usually have the highest caliber of narration, can be found in Appendix B.

The Adventures of Huckleberry Finn
Mark Twain (Samuel Clemens) (1835–1910)

The Adventures of Huckleberry Finn is probably Twain's most enduring work.

RFB&D:	AB FJ152
NLS:	RC 16414
Braille:	BR 3066
Large Print:	APH and Cyber Classics, and North Books sell it; or you can borrow it from the NAVH library
Comm. Aud.:	*Unabridged*: Blackstone, Bookcassette Sales, Books in Motion, Modern Library; *Abridged*: Brilliance Audio, Caedmon (featuring Ed Begley, Jr.), Dove Audio, Durkin Hayes, Penguin Audio (featuring Garrison Keillor), Spoken Arts, Time Warner Audio (study guide)

The Aeneid
Virgil (70–19 B.C.)

The Aeneid is the transition work from Greek culture into Roman, where the story of the fall of Troy is taken up with the journey of the hero Aeneas.

RFB&D:	AB DQ765
NLS:	RC 16338

Braille: BR 10294
Comm. aud.:   Blackstone Audiobooks

Autobiography
Benjamin Franklin (1706–1790)

His *Autobiography* is a thoroughly American story of a man who withdrew indentured servitude and rose through thrift and hard work to become one of the greatest men of his age.

RFB&D: AB TB597
NLS: RC 12633
Braille: BRA 11250
Large print: North Books
Comm. aud.:   *Unabridged*: Audio Partners, Blackstone Audiobooks, Recorded Books

The Autobiography of Malcolm X
Malcolm X (1925–1965)

Alex Haley assisted in the writing of this life story, which traces the rise of Malcolm X from street hustler and convict, through his conversion to Islam, and his rise to prominence in the Black Muslim movement of the 1960s.

RFB&D: AB TB687
NLS: RC 13759
Braille: BR 04416

Battle Cry of Freedom
James McPherson (b. 1936)

Battle Cry of Freedom: The Civil War Era, is considered the best one-volume history of the American Civil War.

RFB&D: AB CC618
NLS: RC 27449

The Bible

The following listings are for the King James version, unabridged.

RFB&D: AB TB580
NLS: RC 40842 (Old Testament) and RC 40843
                (New Testament)
Braille: Available from Bibles for the Blind: 812–
                466–4899
Comm. aud.:   Complete Alexander Scourby reading free on
                web at www.audio-bible.com

The Bluest Eye
Toni Morrison (b. 1931)

Her intricate narratives on the bitter marriage of African women to the American dream and her greatness as a storyteller have made Toni Morrison, who won the 1993 Nobel Prize, one of the best-loved contemporary writers. *The Bluest Eye* is considered one of her best.

RFB&D: AB FH051
NLS: RC 14892
Comm. aud.:   *Abridged*: Random House Audio

A Brief History of Time
Stephen Hawking (b. 1942)

A Brief History of Time covers the origin, history, and fate of the universe in a way that non-physicists can understand.

RFB&D: AB DK195
NLS: RC 31950
Large print: Isis Large Print Books
Comm. aud.:   *Unabridged*: Dove Audio Books

Bury My Heart at Wounded Knee
Dee Brown (b. 1908)

Bury My Heart at Wounded Knee—a classic of history from the Indian perspective.

RFB&D: AB TW827
NLS: RC 20462
Braille: BR 08720

Candide
Voltaire (1694–1778)

The comic masterpiece *Candide, or Optimism* is a hyperbolic dismantling of the notion that we live in the best of all possible worlds.

RFB&D: AB TG501
NLS: RC 31736
Braille: BRA 10107
Large print: APH edition
Comm. aud.:   *Unabridged*: Blackstone Audiobooks, Caedmon

The Canterbury Tales
Geoffrey Chaucer (c. 1340–1400)

Chaucer, like Shakespeare, crystalizes in pure sound the feats and foibles of mankind. His *Canterbury Tales* form the foundation of English literature, with the deepest insights into human character flying forth from a narrative energy that is both humorous and down to earth.

RFB&D: AB TV229
NLS: RC 20461
Braille: BR 466, APH has a 6-volume Braille edition

Large print:	Cyber Classics edition (Thomas T. Beeler, publisher)
Comm. aud.:	H. G. Bissinger's Caedmon Middle English recordings are unsurpassed; a CD-ROM of selections with various readers is available from Audio Books on CD-ROM (www.abcdinc.com)

The Catcher in the Rye
J. D. Salinger (b. 1919)

It is a tale of the breakdown of disaffected Holden Caulfield.

RFB&D:	AB CD351
NLS:	RC 12335
Braille:	BR 01617 (APH also sells braille edition)
Large print:	Little, Brown; NAVH library has circulating copy in 2 volumes

Civil Disobedience
Henry David Thoreau (1817–1862)

Between the philosophical basis of democracy and the sit-ins and protests that marked the 1960s is Thoreau's essay *Civil Disobedience*, which dramatizes a crucial aspect of being American.

RFB&D:	AB AA832
NLS:	RC 15949
Braille:	BR 62
Comm. aud.:	Blackstone Audiobooks, Knowledge Products

Common Sense
Thomas Paine (1737–1809)

Some call America the revolutionary country, and if that is true, the writing that most helped to sustain the effort in the early years was *Common Sense*.

RFB&D: AB TR160
NLS: RC 19603
Braille: BR 32690
Comm. aud.:   Knowledge Products

Confessions
St. Augustine (354–430 A.D.)

The *Confessions* are some of the greatest Christian writings along with the epistles of St. Paul, and the writings of Martin Luther.

RFB&D: AB AQ027
NLS: RC 39444
Comm. aud.:   Blackstone Audiobooks

The Death of Ivan Ilych
Leo Tolstoy (1828–1910)

The Death of Ivan Ilych shows the levels of emotion from understated observations on the highlights of an ordinary man's life.

RFB&D: AB AB892
NLS: RC 09423
Comm. aud.:   Blackstone Audiobooks (includes *Master and Man*)

Democracy in America
Alexis de Tocqueville (1805–1859)

Observing 1830s America, de Tocqueville foresaw a world that would eventually be dominated by the United States and Russia.

RFB&D: AB CA 278
NLS: RC 14244 & 14245
Comm. aud.:   Blackstone Audiobooks

The Divine Comedy
Dante Alighieri (1265–1321)

"There can be only one Dante," said T. S. Eliot. His *Divine Comedy* is among the greatest poems in world literature.

RFB&D:	AB TE047
NLS:	RC 30589
Braille:	BRA 05631
Large print:	Cyber Classics edition (Thomas T. Beeler, publisher)
Comm. aud.:	Buy or rent the complete recording from Blackstone Audiobooks; Penguin Audio offers a new abridgment

A Doll's House
Henrik Ibsen (1828–1906)

A Doll's House, which debuted in 1879, was far ahead of its time in its depiction of a sheltered woman who finds the courage to take flight.

RFB&D:	AB AN699
NLS:	RC 24292
Braille:	BR 06839
Comm. aud.:	Audio Book Contractors

Don Quixote
Miguel de Cervantes Saavedra (1547–1616)

Don Quixote exerted an immense influence on later writers in the Romantic Era, and was a forerunner to the Picaresque and adventure novels that continue to be written today.

RFB&D:	AB TG423
NLS:	RC 24290

Braille: BR 08808
Comm. aud.:   *Unabridged*: Naxos of America (3 CD-ROMs); *Abridged*: Highbridge Company, Dove Audio Books

The Education of Henry Adams
Henry Adams (1838–1918)

The Education of Henry Adams is recognized as one of the greatest autobiographies and treatments of American history ever written.

RFB&D: AB CE551
NLS: RC 22293
Braille: BRA 01119
Comm. aud.:   Blackstone Audiobooks

Essays
Michel de Montaigne (1533–1592)

The personal essay, came about largely due to what Montaigne did with the form in his *Essays*.

RFB&D: AB AL017
NLS: RC 39600
Braille: BRA 07987

An Essay on Man
Alexander Pope (1688–1744)

Pope, like Shakespeare, put lines into our language that are now camouflaged by common usage, such as "To ere is human, to forgive, divine." His *Essay on Man*, is a poetic treatise on mankind.

RFB&D: AB TJ940
NLS: RC 21033

Braille: BRA 18449

Comm. aud.:   The Spoken Art has a *Treasury of Alexander Pope*

Faust
Johann Wolfgang von Goethe (1749–1832)

Faust retells a tale told by Christopher Marlow about a man who sells his soul to the devil, an idea and plot point still popular in todays culture.

RFB&D: AB DL536
NLS: RC 21416
Braille: BRA 15463

The Federalist Papers
Alexander Hamilton (c. 1755–1804), John Jay (1745–1829), James Madison (1751–1836)

Among the greatest political discourses of all time.

RFB&D: AB DM521
NLS: RC 26691
Braille: BRA 04284
Comm. aud.:   Blackstone Audiobooks; also Simon & Schuster's *Giants of Political Thought*, including the "Declaration of Independence" and *Common Sense.*

The Great Gatsby
F. Scott Fitzgerald (1896–1940)

The Great Gatsby is beautifully and sadly American in its portrayal of the destructive power of the illusions wealth brings.

RFB&D: AB FD878
NLS: RC 16147
Braille: BR 11057

Large print: APH and G. K. Hall have editions; NAVH has a circulating copy.

Comm. aud.:   *Unabridged*: Audio Partners, Listening Library (featuring Alexander Scourby), Naxos of America (2 CD-ROMs), Recorded Books; *Abridged*: Durkin Hayes, Naxos of America, Time Warner (study guide), Trafalgar Square

Gulliver's Travels
Jonathan Swift (1667–1745)

Perhaps the greatest satire of the English language written at the height of the age of satire is the novel *Gulliver's Travels*.

RFB&D: AB FJ022

NLS: RC 23150

Braille: BR 2929

Large Print: Cyber Classics edition (Thomas T. Beeler, publisher)

Comm. aud.:   *Unabridged*: Blackstone Audiobooks; *Abridged*: Dove Audio Books (featuring Joel Grey), Highbridge Audio, Penguin Audio, Simon & Schuster (featuring Ted Danson); Time Warner Audio (featuring Stephen Rae)

The History of the Peloponnesian War
Thucydides (c. 460–400 B.C.)

The History of the Peloponnesian War is among the most gripping narratives ever written, recounting in minute and dramatic detail the events of the 27-year war between Athens and Sparta that ended in 404 B.C.

RFB&D: AB AA434

NLS: RC 42452

Braille: BR 10511
Comm. aud.:   Blackstone Audiobooks

I Know Why the Caged Bird Sings
Maya Angelou (b. 1928)

I Know Why the Caged Bird Sings traces Angelou's coming of age in St. Louis.

RFB&D: AB FB924
NLS: RC 24959
Braille: BRA 15299
Comm. aud.:   *Abridged*: Random House Audio (cassette or CD-ROM version)

The Iliad; The Odyssey
Homer (ninth century B.C.)

Homer's epics *The Iliad* and *The Odyssey* detail the end of the Trojan War and Odysseus' long voyage home.

RFB&D: *The Iliad*, AB AM471; *The Odyssey*, AB TE422
NLS: *The Iliad*, RC 09489; *The Odyssey*, RC 14869
Braille: *The Iliad*, BR 09449; *The Odyssey*, BR 05620 (APH sells each in braille)
Large print: Both available in Cyber Classic editions (Thomas T. Beeler, publisher)
Comm. aud.:   Caedmon recordings feature excerpts read by Anthony Quayle; Anton Lesser reads complete *Odyssey* on CD-ROM (www.abcdinc.com)

The Interpretation of Dreams
Sigmund Freud (1856–1939)

The Interpretation of Dreams is a work that helped create psychology.

RFB&D: AB AD576
NLS: RC 09451
Braille: BRA 08426

Leaves of Grass
Walt Whitman (1819–1892)

Whitman was the first truly great American poets. His *Leaves of Grass* opened up free verse techniques that shaped about half the poetry written in this country over the next 155 years.

RFB&D: AB TG934
NLS: RC 32177
Braille: BR 08420 (APH sells 4-volume braille edition)
Comm. aud.:   Blackstone Audiobooks

Lives of Noble Grecians and Romans
Plutarch (c. 46–120 A.D.)

Plutarch's *Lives of the Noble Grecians and Romans*, greatly influenced Shakespeare and Montaigne.

RFB&D: AB FB792 and FB793
NLS: RC 44495
Braille: NLC 006273957
Comm. aud.:   Blackstone Audiobooks

Madame Bovary
Gustave Flaubert (1821–1880)

RFB&D: AB AP600
NLS: RC 13249
Braille: BRA 01999

Comm. aud.:   *Unabridged*: Audio Book Contractors, Audio Partners, Blackstone Audiobooks, and Cover to Cover Cassettes; *Abridged*: Dove Audio, Penguin Audio

Man and His Symbols
Carl Jung (1875–1961)

A bridge between consciousness and unconsciousness is established through an analysis of archetypal symbols in the classic *Man and His Symbols*.

RFB&D: AB TA645
NLS: RC 23876
Braille: BR 007177668
Comm. aud.:   *Abridged*: Audio Scholar, Penton Overseas

Meditations
Marcus Aurelius (121–180 A.D.)

Lines from Marcus Aurelius' *Meditations* are still quoted by today's top motivational experts (e.g. "A man's life is what his thoughts make of it").

RFB&D: AB TF201
NLS: RC 18831
Braille: BRA 15464
Comm. aud.:   Blackstone Audiobooks

The Metamorphoses
Ovid (43 B.C.–A.D. 17)

The *Metamorphoses* collects many stories found in Greek and Roman mythology, such as Phaeton, Niobe, and King Midas.

RFB&D: AB CF613

NLS: RC 26228
Braille: BR 07318

Middlemarch
George Eliot (Mary Ann Evans Cross) (1819–1880)

Many scholars acknowledge *Middlemarch* as one of the greatest novels in the English language.

RFB&D: AB FF931
NLS: RC 20078
Braille: BR 09063
Comm. aud.: *Unabridged*: Audio Book Contractors; *Abridged*: Bantam Audio (BDD radio dramatization), Penguin Audio

Moby Dick
Herman Melville (1819–1891)

Moby Dick is an allegory about an insane sea captain's quest for what he sees as an embodiment of evil.

RFB&D: AB CG613
NLS: RC 34184
Braille: BR 01608
Large print: APH, Cyber Classics edition (Thomas T. Beeler, publisher)
Comm. aud.: *Unabridged*: Audio Books on CD-ROM, Blackstone Audiobooks; *Abridged*: Caedmon (featuring Charlton Heston), Dove Audio (featuring Burt Reynolds), Durkin Hayes (featuring George Kennedy).

Oedipus Rex
Sophocles (c. 496–406 B.C.)

Oedipus Rex has inspired many writers from Aristotle, who used *Oedipus* to define poetry, to Sigmund Freud, who used it to define the nature of the human soul, to Ruth Rendel, who called it one of the mysteries that has always fascinated mankind.

RFB&D:	AB DA962
NLS:	RC 15351
Braille:	BRJ 00884 (Jewish Guild for the Blind)
Comm. aud.:	Caedmon production out of print, but keep checking amazon.com as well as your school and public libraries.

One Day in the Life of Ivan Denisovich
Aleksandr Solzhenitsyn (b. 1918)

In *One Day in the Life of Ivan Denisovich*, a prisoner in a Siberian camp endures one more excruciating day of captivity and finds joy in survival.

RFB&D:	AB FP322
NLS:	RC 18001
Braille:	BRJ 01231
Large print:	Chivers Press
Comm. aud.:	*Unabridged*: Blackstone Audiobooks, Recorded Books

One Hundred Years of Solitude
Gabrial Garcia Marquez (b. 1928)

The twentieth Century saw the emergence of many great Spanish and Latin American poets and writers. Marquez's *One Hundred Years of Solitude* is considered one of the greatest novels written since 1970.

RFB&D:	AB FC656
NLS:	RC 25181
Braille:	BRA 12853
Comm. aud.:	A cassette study guide is available from Time Warner Audio Books

Origin of Species
Charles Darwin (1809–1882)

Darwin did not invent the concept of evolution, but his *Origin of Species*, which advances his theory of natural selection inferred from observations of plant and animal life around the world, gave it disquieting certitude, and forever changed mankind's view of where we came from.

RFB&D:	AB TA400
NLS:	RC 15937
Braille:	BRA 09950
Comm. aud.:	*Abridged*: Audio Scholar, Penton Overseas

Paradise Lost
John Milton (1608–1685)

Milton established himself along with Homer and Virgil as one of the top epic poets in western literature with his poems, notably *Paradise Lost*.

RFB&D:	AB BF827
NLS:	RC 31889
Braille:	BRA 02394
Large print:	Cyber Classics edition (Thomas T. Beeler, publisher)
Comm. aud.:	Blackstone and Naxos Audio Books have it complete; Time Warner Audio offers a 2-cassette study guide

The Pocket Aristotle
Aristotle (384–322 B.C.)

Taught philosophy by Plato, Aristotle went on to master biology, physics, ethics, logic, and poetics, making him the most accomplished thinker of the ancient world. The listings here are for *The Pocket Aristotle*, which includes many of his most famous writings.

RFB&D:	AB TA678
NLS:	RC 44359
Braille:	BRJ 00869 (Jewish Guild for the Blind)
Comm. aud.:	Blackstone Audiobooks sells or rents Aristotle's *Rhetoric, Poetics, and Logic*

The Prince
Niccolo Machiavelli (1469–1527)

The adjective "Machiavellian" occurs in politics and literature all the time.

RFB&D:	AB DQ524
NLS:	RC 39689
Braille:	BRA 09465
Comm. aud.:	*Unabridged*: Audio Partners, Blackstone Audiobooks, Knowledge Products, Penguin Audio

The Red Badge of Courage
Stephen Crane (1871–1900)

Though Crane never set foot on a battlefield, *The Red Badge of Courage* is among the greatest war stories ever written.

RFB&D:	AB TA748
NLS:	RC 22405
Braille:	BR 1449
Large print:	APH edition; or borrow it from NAVH library
Comm. aud.:	*Unabridged*: Blackstone Audiobooks, Bookcassette Sales, Listening Library; *Abridged*: Books in Motion, Brilliance Audio, Dercum Press Audio, Dove Audio (featuring Richard Thomas), Durkin Hayes (featuring Richard Crenna), Metacom, Radio Yesteryear, Random House.

The Republic
Plato (c. 428–348 B.C.)

Through his dialogues, notably his great Utopia *The Republic*, Plato created a system of reasoning that dominated human thought for over 1500 years.

RFB&D: AB TB563
NLS: RC 14875
Braille: NLC 005377275 (Canadian National Institute for the Blind, Toronto)
Comm. aud.:   Blackstone Audiobooks offers unabridged recording

Selected Poems
Emily Dickinson (1830–1886)

All but a handful of Dickinson's poems were published posthumously, and since her death, she has risen straight into the pantheon of world poets.

RFB&D: AB TA692
NLS: RC 23534
Braille: BRA 12518
Comm. aud.:   Julie Harris reads poems and letters for Caedmon; Meryl Streep is featured on *Into the Beautiful*, Time Warner Audio; Sharon Stone et al. read 50 poems for a popular series; Blackstone has a *Selected Poems*.

Selected Works
The Romantic Poets:
William Blake (1757–1827)
William Wordsworth (1770–1850)
Samuel Taylor Coleridge (1772–1834)
Lord George Gordon Byron (1788–1824)

Percy Bysshe Shelley (1792–1822)
John Keats (1795–1821)

In the early nineteenth century, the Romantic movement changed the image of the poet's task from, in Shakespeare's phrase, "holding the mirror up to nature," to, according to M. H. Abrams, adhering to the glow of an inner "lamp" burning within each creative mind.

RFB&D:	AB BA404 (*The Portable Romantic Reader*)
Comm. aud.:	CD-ROM *Great Poets of the Romantic Age* available at www.abcdinc.com

Selected Works
William Shakespeare (1564–1616)

Only the Bible is quoted more than Shakespeare, and no other writer has generated as much scholarship and general reading interest. His plays and poems may be the greatest in any language. They are available in all specialized formats, and are especially powerful in the commercial recordings from Caedmon (often found in libraries) that feature the world's greatest actors.

Sonnets

RFB&D:	AB TA069
NLS:	RC 24580
Braille:	BR 06634

The Tragedy of King Lear

RFB&D:	AB FG648
NLS:	RC 29214
Braille:	BR 1082 & 1525 (APH sells 2-volume braille edition)
Comm. aud.:	CD-ROM version from abcdinc.com

The Tempest

RFB&D:	AB BM156
NLS:	RC 42818
Braille:	BR 1111
Comm. aud.:	CD-ROM version from abcdinc.com

Silent Spring
Rachel Carson (1907–1964)

The environmental and ecological movement, one of the strongest political and social movements of our time, exploded in 1961 with the publication of *Silent Spring*.

RFB&D:	AB TR169
NLS:	RC 20184
Braille:	BR 00210
Comm. aud.:	Durkin Hayes (featuring Ellen Burstyn)

Sound-Shadows of the New World
Ved Mehta (b. 1934)

One of the most accomplished blind writers of our time is *New York Times* columnist Ved Mehta, who chronicles his boyhood displacement from India to rural Arkansas in *Sound-Shadows of the New World*.

NLS:	RD 24156
Braille:	BR 06504

The Stranger
Albert Camus (1913–1960)

Camus, another modern recaster of ancient myths, was the second youngest person to win the Nobel Prize for literature. *The Stranger* was his first and remains his best known novel.

RFB&D:	AB CC381

NLS: RC 40902
Braille: BR 10394 (APH also sells braille edition)

Things Fall Apart
Chinua Achebe (b. 1930)

Things Fall Apart is among the greatest African novels, showing how European influences caused the downfall of a proud village leader.

RFB&D: AB FB 040
Braille: NLC 006758341
Comm. aud.:   *Unabridged*: Recorded Books

Ulysses
James Joyce (1882–1941)

Ulysses traces one day in the lives of three Dubliners, illuminating modern life with ironic points of reference from the chapters of Homer's Odyssey. Caedmon has recordings of Joyce reading one speech, and Milo O'Shea reading the entire first chapter.

RFB&D: AB CE774
NLS: RC 19994
Braille: BR 10287
Comm. aud.:   *Unabridged*: Audiobooks on CD-ROM, Naxos of America (CD-ROM edition): *Abridged*: Caedmon (featuring James Joyce and Milo O'Shea on separate recordings), Penguin Audio

Uncle Tom's Cabin
Harriet Beecher Stowe (1811–1896)

Rarely has an American novel galvanized a movement the way *Uncle Tom's Cabin* did in the 1850s, when it swelled the ranks of the abolitionists, both in the United States and around the world with its portrayal of the evils of slavery.

RFB&D:	AB CD289
NLS:	RC 9480
Braille:	BR 1623
Large print:	APH has 2-volume edition
Comm. aud.:	*Unabridged*: Blackstone Audiobooks; *Abridged*: Bookcassette Sales, Brilliance Audio

Up from Slavery
Booker T. Washington (1856–1915)

Few people in American history began as low and rose as high as Booker T. Washington, who was born a slave, and later became one of the most influential educators and advocates on social justice.

RFB&D:	AB TC084
NLS:	RC 32540
Braille:	BR 09609
Comm. aud.:	Blackstone Audiobooks

The Waste Land
T. S. Eliot (1888–1965)

The Waste Land is one of the most significant poems of the twentieth century. This listing below is for the *Collected Poems*.

RFB&D:	AB BK129
NLS:	RC 19566
Braille:	BRA 02624
Comm. aud.:	Caedmon (featuring T. S. Eliot), Penguin Audio (featuring Ted Hughes)

The Wealth of Nations
Adam Smith (1723–1790)

The Wealth of Nations is still one of the seminal works in economics, a discipline that Americans have come to dominate in the twentieth century.

RFB&D: AB AC697
NLS: RC 23688
Braille: BRA 08707
Comm. aud.:   *Unabridged*: Blackstone Audiobooks; *Abridged*: Knowledge Products

RESOURCES

American Library Association
50 East Huron Street
Chicago, IL 60611
Phone: 800–545–2433
Internet: www.ala.org

Books that Changed the World
by Robert B. Downs
New York: Penguin Books, 1983

RFB&D: AB BW986
NLS: RC 33153
Braille: BR 8730

Great Books Foundation
35 East Wacker Drive
Suite 2300
Chicago, IL 60601–2298
Phone: 800–222–5870
Internet: www.greatbooks.org

Appendix D: The Americans with Disabilities Act in the Library

No book promoting opportunities for the sight-impaired would be complete without mentioning the Americans with Disabilities Act (Public Law 101–336), which President George Bush signed into law on July 26, 1990. Described by some as the Emancipation Proclamation for America's 43 million disabled citizens, the ADA prohibits discrimination and ensures equal opportunity for persons with disabilities in employment, state and local government services, public accommodations, commercial facilities, and transportation. It also mandates the establishment of TDD/telephone relay services.

The law is so important that all sight-impaired readers and those who serve them should understand its provisions. The ADA will not force a library to automatically relocate a book discussion group to a more accessible place, nor provide a sign language interpreter to a children's story hour. However, when such requests are made in advance, the library should make every effort to accommodate you. Thus the ADA can help you develop the crucial habit of determining what you need and want from a library. It also provides a platform of courage that may make asking easier for you.

In general, libraries will make changes that will benefit the largest number of patrons. For example, instead of supplying you with a live reader, your librarian might obtain funds for a closed-circuit TV or a computer equipped with screen reading software—items that might serve many needs within the community.

There are requirements that libraries must follow when making significant renovations or expansions. These are strict structural guidelines that affect the creation of reading and study areas, stacks, and reference rooms; card catalog placement; reserve areas; checkout; and book security gates.

For what sight-impaired readers need, most librarians are eager to lend a hand.

AMERICANS WITH DISABILITIES ACT RESOURCES

The complete text of the Americans with Disabilities Act, Public Law 101–336, can be obtained in braille and on cassette for free from the American Printing House for the Blind (see Chapter 2) or the National Library Service affiliate in your state (see Appendix A). A solid book on the ADA and its provisions is *Complying with the Americans with Disabilities Act: A Guidebook for Management and People with Disabilities*, by Don Fersh, which is available from Recording for the Blind & Dyslexic (Shelf# AB FK982).

Title I: Employment Issues

Equal Opportunity Employment Commission
Room 9024
1801 L Street NW

Washington, DC 20507
Toll free: 800–669–4000 (questions); 800–669–3362 (literature requests)

Publications:

The ADA Handbook

The ADA—Your Employment Rights as an Individual with a Disability

Title I Technical Assistance Manual

Title I Regulations, 29 CFR Parts 1502, 1627, and 1630, Equal Employment Opportunity for Individuals with Disabilities, Final Rule

Title II and Title III: Transportation Issues

Department of Transportation
400 Seventh Street SW
Washington, DC 20590
Phone: 202–366–1656 (general questions and literature requests); 202–366–1936 (legal questions)

Publication:

Title II and Title III Regulations, 49 CFR Parts 27, 37, and 38, Transportation for Individuals with Disabilities, Final Rule.

Title II and Title III: Government, Public Accommodations, and Commercial Facility Issues

Disability Rights Section
Civil Rights Division
U.S. Department of Justice
PO Box 66738

Washington, DC 20035–6738
Toll free: 800–514–0301

Publications:

Title II Highlights

Title II Technical Assistance Manual

Title II Regulations, 28 CFR Part 35, Nondiscrimination on the Basis of Disability in State and Local Government Services, Final Rule

Title III Highlights

Title III Technical Assistance Manual

Title III Regulations, 28 CFR Part 36, Nondiscrimination on the Basis of Disability by Public Accommodations and in Commercial Facilities, Final Rule

Title III Requirements in Public Accommodations Fact Sheet

Accessible Design

Architectural and Transportation Barriers Compliance Board
The Access Board
1331 F Street NW Suite 1000
Washington, DC 20004
Phone: 202–272–5434
Toll free: 800–872–2253

Publications:

Title II and III Guidelines, 36 CFR Part 1191, Accessibility Guidelines for Buildings and Facilities, Final Guidelines

Title II and III Guidelines, 36 CFR Part 1191, Accessibility Guidelines for Buildings and Facilities and Transportation, Final Guidelines

Title II and III Guidelines, 36 CFR Part 1192, Accessibility Guidelines for Transportation Vehicles, Final Guidelines

Appendix E: Grant Sources for Funding ADA Projects in the Library

Julie Klauber, an outreach services librarian and president of Disability Resources, got grant funding for her nonprofit organization's newsletter—which circulates for free to over 2,000 libraries—from the Paralyzed Veterans of America Spinal Cord Injury Education and Training Foundation. Though hard to find, and demanding great creativity and patience to pursue, funding opportunities do exist for the librarian to upgrade services, collections, and equipment, whether to comply with the ADA or to enhance existing programs.

Since adaptive computer technology is becoming central to the sight-impaired reader's life, enhanced reading opportunities might be gained by adding computers equipped with screen readers, or that use closed-circuit TV as the monitor for enlarging text. Seeing if you qualify for a grant under the Library Services and Technology Act (administered through your state library system) might be the place to start.

There is a chance that federal block grants for ADA compliance may still be available. This is tough, since the law is nearly a decade old. Information on state and municipal grants is often difficult to find. Check with local government officials and congressional offices to see what information they have. Federal funders generally prefer projects that serve as prototypes or models for others to replicate; local government funders require strong evidence of community support for a project. Government grants nearly always have strict reporting requirements. Careful record keeping is a must, since an audit is always a possibility. Government funding programs and priorities change frequently, so it is a good idea to call the agency in question before applying for funding in order to obtain the most up-to-date information on its programs.

The following list of publications and websites might be useful in seeking government funding.

Government Assistance Almanac
By J. Robert Dumouchel
Detroit, MI: Omnigraphics, annual

www.gsa.gov/fdac/default.htm
The Catalog of Federal Domestic Assistance
This is a searchable database of information about federal assistance programs.

web.fie.com/fedix/index.html
FEDIX
This database of federal funding opportunities is searchable by agency, audience, and subject. Visitors may sign up for E-mail funding opportunity updates.

www.nonprofit.gov
The Nonprofit Gateway
This website includes links to federal websites and information about grant programs, arranged by cabinet department and federal agency. Visitors can search Notices of Funding Availability from the *Federal Register*.

FOUNDATION GRANTS

A good place to begin fund-raising research for foundation grants is with the FAQ topics located in the Online Library section of the Foundation Center website, especially the FAQ "How do I find out about grants for my subject area or field of interest?" The Online Library also offers a self-guided orientation, providing a more in-depth introduction to the grant-seeking and funding research process. The site also contains a Grantmaker Information section with which you can begin searching for potential foundation funders on the Internet right away. A Grantmaker Search feature on the same site enables you to search abstracts describing foundation websites by subject or geographic area.

While at present only a few foundations use the web to make their guidelines known, that number is growing daily. Another site worth a look is the Community Foundation Locator at the Council on Foundations (www.cof.org/community), which can tell you whether there is a foundation serving your local area.

Here are two more resources:

National Guide to Funding in Health
New York: The Foundation Center
This book can be viewed for free at over 200 cooperating libraries and the five Foundation Centers. Its index contains many entries on blindness and related issues.

FC Search Database on CD-ROM, Version 2.1
New York: The Foundation Center
Combines numerous Foundation Center publications with powerful search capabilities.

Selected Bibliography

American Foundation for the Blind. *AFB Directory of Services for Blind and Visually Impaired Persons in the United States and Canada*, 25th ed. New York: AFB Press, 1997.

Castellano, Carol, and Dawn Kosman. *The Bridge to Braille: Reading and School Success for the Young Blind Child.* Baltimore, MD: National Federation of the Blind, 1997.

Fersh, Don, and Peter W. Thomas. *Complying with the Americans with Disabilities Act: A Guidebook for Management and People with Disabilities.* Westport, CT: Greenwood Publishing Group, 1993.

Jahoda, Gerald. *How Do I Do This When I Can't See What I'm Doing?: Information Processing for the Visually Disabled.* Washington, DC: Library of Congress, 1993.

Jernigan, Kenneth, ed. *If Blindness Comes.* Baltimore, MD: National Federation of the Blind, 1994.

Jernigan, Kenneth, ed. *What You Should Know about Blindness, Services for the Blind, and the Organized Blind Movement.* Baltimore, MD: National Federation of the Blind, 1992.

Majeska, Marilyn Lundell. *Talking Books: Pioneering and Beyond.* Washington, DC: Library of Congress, 1988.

McNulty, Tom, and Dawn M. Suvino. *Access to Information: Materials, Technologies, and Services for Print-Impaired Readers.* Washington, DC: American Library Association, 1993.

National Library Service for the Blind and Physically Handi-
    capped; Library Resources for the Blind and Physically
    Handicapped. A Directory of FY 1997 Statistics on
    Readership Circulation, Budget, Staff, and Collections.
    Washington, DC: Library of Congress, 1997.
Rex, Evelyn J., Alan J. Koenig, Diane P. Wormsley, and Robert
    L. Baker. *Foundations of Braille Literacy*. New York:
    American Foundation for the Blind, 1995.
Sardegna, Jill, and T. Otis Paul. *The Encyclopedia of Blindness
    and Visual Impairment*. New York: Facts on File, 1991.
Younger, Vivian, and Jill Sardegna. *A Guide to Independence
    for the Visually Impaired and Their Families*. New
    York: Demos Vermande, 1994.

Index

About the Author

ANDREW LEIBS is an award-winning writer of over 2000 newspaper and magazine pieces that have appeared in such publications as *Dialogue* and *The San Francisco Examiner*.